Cardiac CT Made Easy

Cardiac CT Made Easy

An Introduction to Cardiovascular Multidetector Computed Tomography

Third Edition

Edited by

Paul Schoenhagen MD
Imaging Institute and Heart & Vascular Institute
Cleveland Clinic
Cleveland, Ohio

Frank Dong PhD, DABR, FAAPM
Imaging Institute, Section of Medical Physics
Cleveland Clinic
Cleveland, Ohio

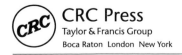
CRC Press
Taylor & Francis Group
Boca Raton London New York

CRC Press is an imprint of the
Taylor & Francis Group, an **informa** business

Third edition published 2023
by CRC Press
6000 Broken Sound Parkway NW, Suite 300, Boca Raton, FL 33487-2742

and by CRC Press
4 Park Square, Milton Park, Abingdon, Oxon, OX14 4RN

CRC Press is an imprint of Taylor & Francis Group, LLC

Library of Congress Cataloging-in-Publication Data

Names: Schoenhagen, Paul, editor. | Dong, Frank, editor. Title: Cardiac CT made easy : an introduction to cardiovascular multidetector computed tomography / edited by Paul Schoenhagen, Frank Dong.
Description: Third edition. | Boca Raton, FL : CRC Press, Taylor & Francis, 2022. | Includes bibliographical references and index. | Summary: "Cardiovascular Computed Tomography has a prominent role in the diagnosis and management across a wide spectrum of clinical indications. With a focus on visual material, the 3rd edition has been carefully revised and updated to include recent developments in CT scanner technology and clinical indications for imaging specialists and clinicians"-- Provided by publisher. Identifiers: LCCN 2022015561 (print) | LCCN 2022015562 (ebook) | ISBN 9780367721480 (hardback) | ISBN 9780367721473 (paperback) | ISBN 9781003153641 (ebook) Subjects: MESH: Cardiovascular Diseases--diagnostic imaging | Tomography, X-Ray Computed--methods | Atlas Classification: LCC RC670 (print) | LCC RC670 (ebook) | NLM WG 17 | DDC 616.1/075--dc23/eng/20220412 LC record available at https://lccn.loc.gov/2022015561LC ebook record available at https://lccn.loc.gov/2022015562

ISBN: 9780367721480 (hbk)
ISBN: 9780367721473 (pbk)
ISBN: 9781003153641 (ebk)

DOI: 10.1201/9781003153641

Typeset in Minion
by KnowledgeWorks Global Ltd.

Printed in the UK by Severn, Gloucester on responsibly sourced paper

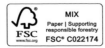

Contents

Foreword

Driven by constant technical improvement, cardiac Computed Tomography (CT) continues to find ever broader applications in cardiology. From cardiovascular disease prevention to the management of patients with suspected coronary artery disease, from the support of electrophysiology procedures to coronary and structural interventions, and from the emergency room to specialized clinics: many areas of cardiovascular care benefit from the capability of cardiac CT to provide high-resolution anatomic and functional information. There is no doubt that contemporary cardiology practice relies heavily on the imaging information provided by CT and most certainly, applications of CT imaging in cardiovascular medicine will continue to grow.

New CT technology, optimized acquisition protocols, dedicated image reconstruction algorithms, and advanced image processing methods have introduced both increased applicability, but also somewhat added complexity to cardiac CT. This is why the third edition of *Cardiac CT Made Easy* comes at the right time. Written by clinical experts with enormous experience, the book follows a clear and concise style and comprehensively covers all relevant areas of coronary and vascular disease, heavily illustrated by representative images.

I would like to thank and congratulate the authors for the creation of this most welcome third edition and for their contribution to the field. Readers across the world will benefit from the clinically relevant information that is provided in such a succinct form. Ultimately, the book will contribute to the further development of cardiac and vascular CT to enhance the care of countless patients.

Stephan Achenbach, MD, FESC, FACC, MSCCT
Professor of Medicine
University of Erlangen
Erlangen, Germany

Editors

Paul Schoenhagen MD, is Professor of Radiology at Case Western University, Cleveland Clinic Lerner College of Medicine. He is a staff physician in the Department of Diagnostic Radiology and in the Department of Cardiovascular Medicine. His clinical interest is focused on cardiovascular imaging with computed tomography and magnetic resonance imaging. He received his initial clinical training in internal medicine and radiology in Stuttgart, Germany. This was followed by a residency in internal medicine and fellowships in cardiology and in cardiovascular tomography at Cleveland Clinic. Dr Schoenhagen was appointed to Cleveland Clinic in 2003. He has published numerous original and review articles in leading peer-reviewed journals. He has been invited to present his clinical experience and research at medical symposia and conferences in Japan, China, Europe, and nationally.

Frank Dong PhD, DABR, FAAPM, is a staff diagnostic physicist and an Associate Professor of Radiology at the Cleveland Clinic. Dr Dong received his PhD in medical physics from the University of Wisconsin-Madison. Dr Dong's specialty is in the field of CT image quality, CT radiation dosimetry, and diagnostic ultrasound. He has authored and co-authored 38 peer-reviewed articles, 3 book chapters, 15 patents, and 88 national and international meeting abstracts/presentations. His clinical research is focused on low contrast lesion detectability with advanced CT reconstruction algorithms, as well as the impact of metal artefact reduction on low contrast lesion detection using custom-designed arthroplasty phantom. Dr Dong is the co-investigator of an industrially funded research project involving evaluation of image quality and diagnostic efficacy of a photon counting CT (PCCT). He currently serves as the Director for the American Association of Physicists in Medicine (AAPM) Diagnostic Review Courses. He also serves as the AAPM representative to the writing group of the American College of Radiology (ACR)–AAPM Technical Standard for CT Performance Monitoring. Dr Dong is a Fellow of AAPM, a member of the American College of Radiology, and the Intersocietal Accreditation Commission (IAC) CT Board of Directors.

Contributors

Lei Zhao MD
Department of Radiology
Beijing Anzhen Hospital
Capital Medical University
Beijing, China

Xiaohai Ma MD, PhD
Department of Radiology
Beijing Anzhen Hospital
Capital Medical University
Beijing, China

Section 1

Basics of Multidetector Computed Tomography (MDCT)

Introduction to Cardiovascular MDCT Imaging

The diagnostic use of computed tomography (CT) is based on seminal developments in the field of physics during the 1970s.[1,2] Since then, CT has matured into an established diagnostic imaging modality across multiple specialties and has witnessed an exponential increase in use.[3] In cardiovascular medicine, newer generations of scanner technology have expanded the diagnostic spectrum to include assessment of the large vessels (aorta, pulmonary artery), myocardium, pericardium, cardiac valves, and coronary arteries. CT is used in the initial diagnosis, treatment planning for standard or minimally invasive cardiothoracic surgery and transcatheter interventions, and disease follow-up.[4]

Since the publication of the first edition of this book, almost two decades ago in 2006, knowledge about this imaging modality has become ever more important for imaging specialists and clinicians alike. This book is developed for readers from multiple clinical specialties, who are learning about cardiovascular CT. It is intended to be a short practical introduction with a focus on visual material, complementary to more detailed textbooks.[5]

The book describes the principles of multidetector computed tomography (MDCT) for cardiovascular applications, practical aspects of scan acquisition and interpretation, clinical indications and imaging protocols, and clinical findings of common cardiovascular disease conditions. The comparison with other imaging modalities, such as conventional angiography, intravascular ultrasound, magnetic resonance imaging, and echocardiography, allows understanding of the strength and limitations of CT in the assessment of specific clinical questions.

The basic concept of CT is the reconstruction of thin image slices from multiple projections obtained by rotating an X-ray source and detector system around the patient. In the resulting *tomographic* image, individual structures are differentiated by different image intensities (Hounsfield units). The acquired slices from the entire covered scan range (z-coverage) are combined into a three-dimensional (3-D) volume, which can be reconstructed along unlimited oblique planes following the data acquisition using dedicated computer workstations.

The advantages of tomographic CT imaging are partially offset by the lower temporal resolution (longer time required to obtain data) compared to e.g. angiography. Because of the rapid, constant motion of the heart during the cardiac cycle, long acquisition times increase cardiac motion artefact (image blurring). The development of dedicated cardiovascular CT systems therefore required optimization of acquisition times and synchronization of imaging acquisition with the cardiac cycle.

This was initially realized with electron-beam technology (EBCT),[6] but these scanners were subsequently replaced by MDCT. In MDCT systems, the gantry (X-ray tube and detector) rotates rapidly around the patient (**Figure 1.1**). Initial single detector CT systems, introduced in 1972 for body imaging, were limited by very slow rotation and long acquisition time. Fast gantry rotation, thin collimated detector rows, ECG-synchronized imaging, and acquisition

DOI: 10.1201/9781003153641-2

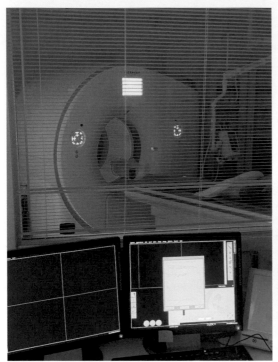
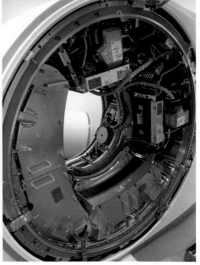

Figure 1.1 Multidetector CT technology (MDCT). A third-generation dual-source scanner, photographed from the "control-room" (top panel), and with open cover showing the gantry (bottom panel).

of multiple slices per gantry rotation have since allowed the development of modern cardiovascular systems.[7,8] Dual-source scanners, with two X-ray tubes/detector systems were introduced in 2008, and allowed a 50% reduction in temporal resolution.[9] Today, high-end scanners permit rotation times as low as 250 ms, with resulting temporal resolution of 135 ms (single source) and 66 ms (dual source). Modern systems acquire up to 320 slices per rotation with a minimum collimated detector row width of 0.5 or 0.625 mm resulting in isotropic spatial resolution below 0.5 mm.

CT Perspective of Normal Cardiovascular Anatomy

Because of the oblique orientation of the cardiovascular structures in the chest, cardiovascular imaging depends on acquisition or reconstructions of defined standard image planes oblique to the body axes ('z-axis'). These include e.g. two-, three-, and four-chamber views of the left ventricle (LV) and are well known from e.g. echocardiography. With two-dimensional (2-D) imaging modalities (e.g. standard echocardiography, most magnetic resonance sequences, and standard angiography), these image planes are obtained at the time of image acquisition and cannot be modified at the time of review. For 3-D modalities (computed tomography, 3-D echocardiography, 3-D magnetic resonance imaging [MRI] sequences, and rotational angiography) a 3-D data volume is acquired and oblique planes are reconstructed at the time of image analysis at the workstation. The ability to reconstruct the data volume in unlimited oblique planes is one of the strengths of CT and other 3-D modalities.

The image processing techniques most often used are 2-D multiplanar reformation (MPR) and maximum intensity projection (MIP), 3-D shaded surface display (SSD) and volume rendering (VR), and 4-D volume rendering.[10] The quality of these reformatted images depends on the in-plane and through-plane spatial resolution. If the through-plane resolution or slice thickness is less than the in-plane resolution of axial images, oblique reformation will be associated with a loss of spatial resolution compared with axial images. It is also important to understand that advanced 3-D and 4-D displays of the CT data can be associated with loss of image detail. Therefore, experienced CT readers typically form their initial impression using the axial 'source' images and then supplement the review with advanced 3-D images.

2.1 Axial CT Images

Because CT systems acquire data in the axial plane, these images have the highest spatial resolution. Therefore, the initial step for the interpretation of CT images remains review of the individual tomographic axial image slices. Experienced readers are able to gain a 3-D understanding from this review.

2.1.1 Two-Dimensional Reformation

The strength of volumetric 3-D CT imaging is that image processing allows reformation in unlimited planes not specified at the time of data acquisition. This is critically important for cardiac imaging, because most cardiac axes are oblique to the axial plane. Interactive computer

DOI: 10.1201/9781003153641-3

workstations allow the user to place orthogonal planes through the data set, creating sagittal and coronal images. Further manipulation of the reformatted plane provides oblique images following the orientation of cardiac structures, e.g. the LV or the aortic root. In addition, curved planes that follow the course of tortuous vessels, e.g. the coronary arteries, can be created automatically or by tracing the path of the vessel on the original axial images. The resulting curved image displays the 3-D course of the vessel. However, the surrounding anatomy is sometimes distorted in these images.

The axial 'source' image is a 2-D grey-scale image displaying all pixels in an individual image slice with a given slice thickness chosen during image reconstruction. 2-D images can be reconstructed in different formats at an arbitrary slice thickness. The simplest image processing method for visualization is MPR. An MPR is a 2-D image displaying all pixels in a chosen plane. The original CT values are preserved. Therefore, in a contrast-enhanced MPR image, e.g. of a coronary vessel, both the high-intensity signal of the contrast-filled lumen and the low-intensity signal of the vessel wall are represented. Another common reconstruction technique is the MIP. In contrast to the MPR, the MIP is a 2-D image displaying only the maximum-intensity pixels. Therefore, in a contrast-enhanced MIP image of the coronary vessel, visualization of the lumen is optimized, but the wall structures are not well seen. Because of their similarity to conventional angiograms, MIP images are often used for CT angiography. However, only a part of the original CT data are preserved, and specifically changes of the vessel wall including atherosclerotic plaque may be missed.

2.1.2 Three-Dimensional Reformation

Volume-rendered (VR) techniques employ advanced 3-D image processing algorithms with semitransparent visualization of superficial and deep contours. Each voxel is assigned a value for opacity according to its CT number, such that lower-intensity tissues are more transparent while higher-intensity tissues are more opaque. Therefore, the more opaque tissue is visible through translucent tissue, creating depth perception. VR images allow the demonstration of complex anatomy and appreciation of the spatial relationship between visualized structures. Levels of opacity can be varied to alter the display of data as needed. In addition, the VR data can be viewed at arbitrary angles, including the standard views of conventional coronary angiography (right anterior oblique/ left anterior oblique [RAO/LAO], cranial/caudal). Colour coding can also be used to enhance further the 3-D appearance.

Perspective volume rendering (pVR) provides virtual endoscopic views of the surface of anatomic structures that are sufficiently contrasted from surrounding tissue.[11] This technique is used to visualize cavities or tubular structures accessible to endoscopes (e.g. the colon or the bronchial tree). Although the clinical value is unclear, pVR can also be applied to chambers of the heart or vascular structures, which can be viewed from within the lumen.

2.1.3 Dynamic, '4-Dimensional' Reconstruction

Retrospective ECG-gated spiral techniques and, to a more limited extent prospective ECG-triggered sequential techniques on some systems, allow reconstruction of data for functional assessment (e.g. ejection fraction calculation). Multiple image sets from different phases in the cardiac cycle are reconstructed and combined into a cine loop to produce a dynamic image set. These images allow qualitative assessment of, e.g. left ventricular function, and dynamic visualization of the complete spatial 3-D data set (4-D imaging). It is important to remember that these dynamic data sets reflect data from only one or two heartbeats and therefore do not allow beat-to-beat assessment, which is a strength of echocardiography. Further, the temporal resolution is inferior to echocardiography and in particular thin, highly mobile structures are expected to be better visualized with echocardiography.

2.1.3.1 Cardiac chambers

The left and right cardiac chambers are visualized in two-chamber, three-chamber, four-chamber, and short-axis views (**Figure 2.1**).

- The two-chamber view of the LV is comparable to the RAO ventriculogram performed during angiography (**Figure 2.2**). In contrast to angiography, CT (also MRI, and echocardiography) visualize both the contrast-filled ventricular cavity and the myocardial wall.
- The three-chamber view includes the left atrium, LV, and aortic root. It visualizes the relationship between the LV, mitral valve, and left ventricular outflow tract (LVOT) (**Figure 2.3**, left upper panel). It is also the basis to reconstruct additional images of the aortic and mitral annulus

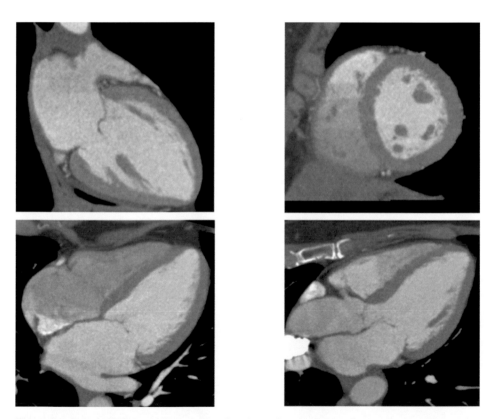

Figure 2.1 Standard views of the cardiac chambers. Standard planes for visualization of the cardiac chamber are two-chamber (left upper panel), three-chamber (right lower panel), four-chamber (left lower panel), and short-axis (right upper panel) views.

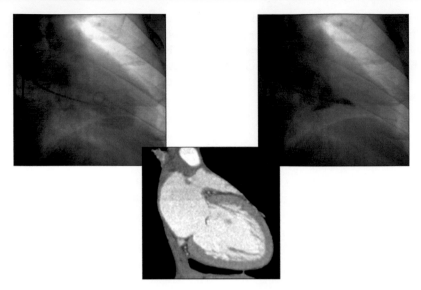

Figure 2.2 Two-chamber view. The two-chamber view is comparable to the left ventriculogram in the RAO projection, performed during angiography. The CT two-chamber view of the LV (lower panel) visualizes both the contrast-filled ventricular cavity and the myocardial wall.

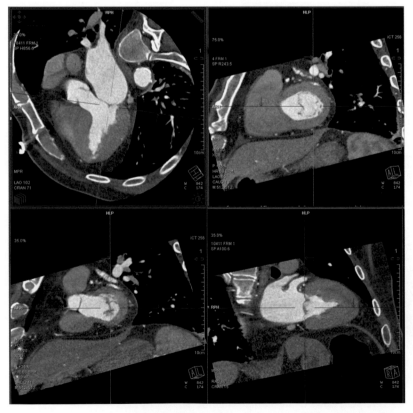

Figure 2.3 Three-chamber view. A typical three-chamber is shown in the left upper panel. The short-axis view shows the mitral valve in diastole (right upper panel) and systole (left lower panel).

- The four-chamber view allows simultaneous assessment of left and right ventricles (LV and RV), the atria (LA and RA), and the atrioventricular valves (mitral and tricuspid valve) (**Figure 2.4**, left upper panel). Quantification of left and right ventricular function is possible if data is acquired throughout the entire cardiac cycle (retrospective gating) and reconstructed at end diastole and end systole.[12]

2.1.3.2 Central venous and pulmonary venous return

- Venous return from the upper and lower parts of the body drains via the superior vena cava (SVC) and inferior vena cava IVC) drain into the right atrium (**Figure 2.5**). The SVC and IVC extend in a cranial-caudal orientation. Therefore, simple review of the axial images provides near cross-sectional images, frequently without need for additional 3-D reconstructions.
- The coronary venous blood flow drains via the coronary sinus into the RA (**Figure 2.6**). It originates at the inferior-medical aspect of the RA, and bifurcates into branches extending parallel to the coronary arteries. The largest branch lies inferior to the LA, and then extends as the great cardiac vein along the left AV groove (along the left circumflex

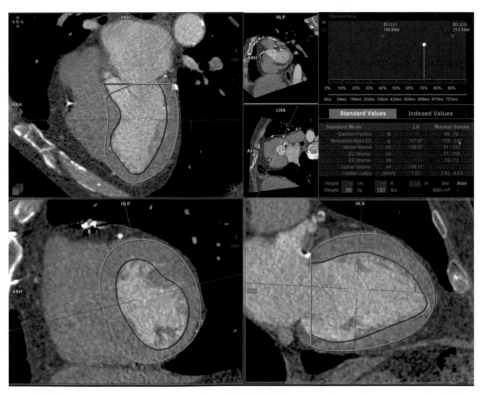

Figure 2.4 Four-chamber view. The four-chamber view (left upper panel) allows simultaneous assessment of left and right ventricle, atria, and atrioventricular valves (mitral and tricuspid valve). If the CT images are acquired in different phases of the cardiac cycle (retrospective gating), data reconstruction allows display of systolic and diastolic images for functional analysis. Modern software allows automatic segmentation of the LV/RV cavity. In this figure, LV endocardial and epicardial borders are identified. This allows calculation of ejection fraction, LV volumes, and myocardial mass, as demonstrated in this figure.

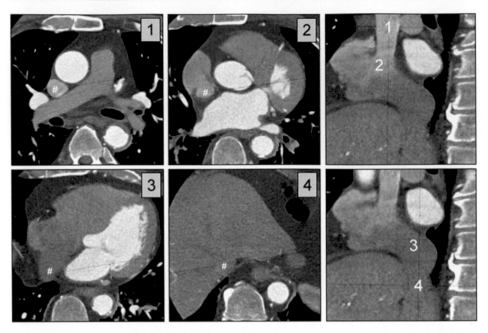

Figure 2.5 Central venous return – SVC and IVC. The superior and inferior vena cava drain into the right atrium. Because the SVC and IVC are extended in a cranial-caudal orientation, review of the axial images provides near cross-sectional images, frequently without the need for additional 3-D reconstructions. This figure shows axial images at several levels in the SVC and IVC and the location in a sagittal image.

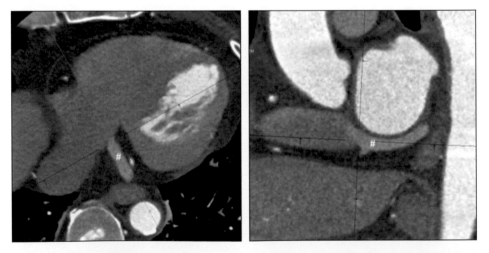

Figure 2.6 Coronary sinus. The coronary sinus (asterisk) drains the coronary flow into the right atrium. This figure shows the close relationship to the left atrium.

artery [LCX]) to the anterior interventricular groove (parallel to the left anterior descending artery [LAD]).

- Venous return from the lungs drains via the pulmonary veins into the LA. Each lung lobe has separate drainage, which merge centrally. There are typically two left veins, the

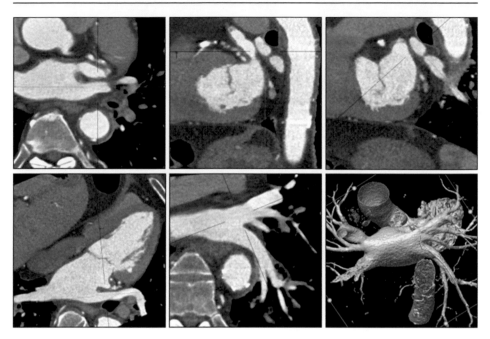

Figure 2.7 Pulmonary veins. Venous return from the lungs drains via the pulmonary veins into the left atrium. The upper left and upper middle panels show axial and sagittal images with the cross-hair centred on the left superior vein. In the upper right panel, the planes are tilted through the left upper and lower veins, resulting in an oblique axial image showing both veins (lower middle panel). The lower right panel shows a volume-rendered image of the pulmonary veins.

left superior and left inferior and the left lingua lobar branch typically originates from the left superior vein. Frequently there is a common antrum or stem of the left veins. In most patients there are two right veins, the right superior and the right inferior vein. The right middle lobe vein is typically a branch of the right superior vein and less frequently drains separately into the LA. Initial review in axial and sagittal images provides a good overview. If necessary, dedicated reconstructions along individual veins can be obtained and also visualized with volume-rendered images (VRIs) (**Figure 2.7**).

2.1.3.3 Pulmonary artery

The RV connects via the right ventricular outflow tract (RVOT) with the pulmonary artery (PA). The pulmonary valve lies at the transition between the RVOT and PA. The normal pulmonary valve is typically not well seen due to the thin, mobile leaflets. The central PA bifurcates into the right and left main vessels before further branching in the lungs (**Figure 2.8**). Depending on the timing of the contrast bolus, the vascular tree with smaller segmental and sub-segmental branches is visualized.

2.1.3.4 Aorta

2.1.3.4.1 Aortic root

The aortic root is a transition zone between the LVOT and tubular ascending aorta.

- The anatomic transition between the LVOT (**Figure 2.9**) and root is the crown-shaped insertion of the aortic valve leaflets. By imaging, the aortic annulus/annular plane is defined by the lowest insertion point of the aortic valve leaflets (**Figure 2.9**). Precise measurement

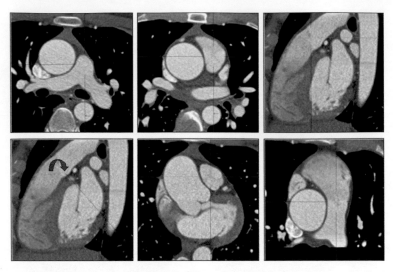

Figure 2.8 Pulmonary artery. The pulmonary valve lies at the transition between the RVOT and PA. The central pulmonary artery bifurcates into the right and left main vessels before further branching in the lungs. This figure shows axial (upper left and upper middle) and sagittal images (upper right) of the central pulmonary artery. In the lower panels, oblique images are reconstructed at the level of the pulmonary valve.

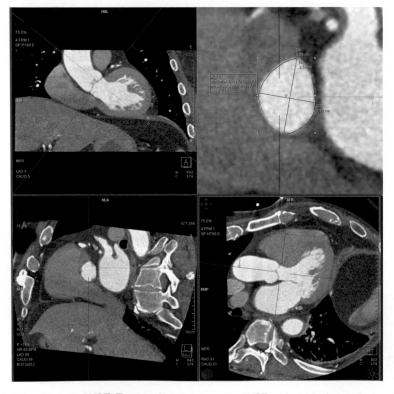

Figure 2.9 Aortic root, LVOT. The transition between the LVOT and root is the aortic annulus. The annulus anatomically has the shape of a crown. By imaging, the 'annular plane' is defined by the lowest insertion point of the aortic valves. Precise measurement of the aortic annulus with minimal and maximal diameter, circumference, and area is critically important for the evaluation in the context of TAVR.

of the minimal and maximal diameter, circumference, and area is critically important for the evaluation in the context of transcatheter aortic valve replacement (TAVR).

- At the aortic valve, the left-, right-, and non-coronary cusp can be differentiated. In retrospective gated studies, images can be reconstructed with the valve open (systole) and closed (diastole) and opening area can be assessed (**Figure 2.10**).
- Around the aortic valve level, there is mild physiologic bulging in the area of the sinuses of Valsalva (**Figure 2.11**). The sinuses correspond to the three aortic valve cusps including the non-coronary cusp (the cusp originating between left and right atria), and the right and left coronary cusps with the origin of the corresponding coronary arteries. Aortic root measurements are made at the level of the maximum diameter of the sinuses of Valsalva (**Figure 2.11**).
- The segment between the sinuses of Valsalva and ascending aorta is called the sinotubular junction (STJ) and typically causes a mild waist.

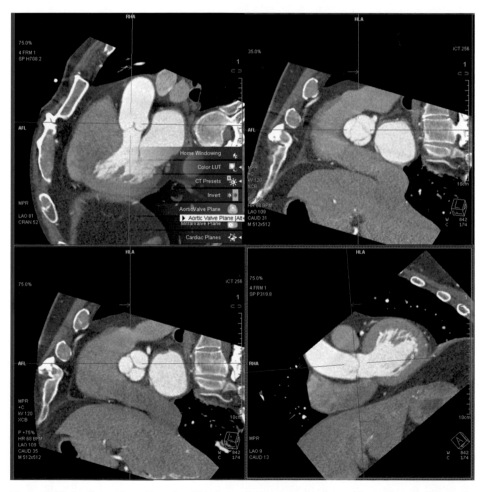

Figure 2.10 Aortic root, aortic valve. This figure shows reconstructions of the aortic root at the aortic valve level. Cross-sectional images are reconstructed in systole (right upper panel) and diastole (left lower panel). The cross-hair in the left upper and right lower panel demonstrates the location of the cross-sectional reconstruction.

13

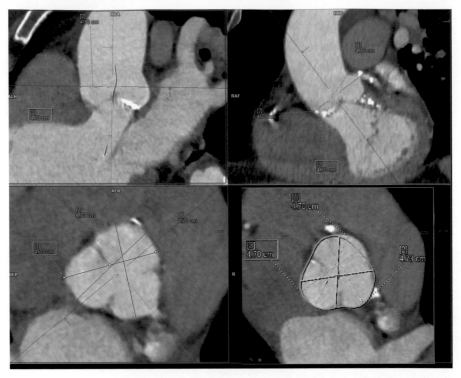

Figure 2.11 Aortic root, diameter measurement at the sinuses of Valsalva. The images in this figure show diameter measurements of the aortic root at the level of the sinuses of Valsalva. Reconstruction of the aortic root also allows identifying the origin of the coronary arteries relative to the cusps of the aortic root.

2.1.3.4.2 Thoracic and abdominal aortic segments

The anatomy of the tubular aorta is reconstructed along the centreline of the vessel, with longitudinal and cross-sectional images. This can be done by manual reconstruction or semi-automated centreline reconstructions (**Figure 2.12**). The aorta is divided into several segments. Beyond the aortic root, these segments include:

- Ascending aorta
- Aortic arch with the ostia of the arch branch vessels
- Descending aorta
- Juxtarenal aorta with the origin of the arch branch vessels
- Infrarenal aorta and the iliac arteries

2.1.3.5 Coronary arteries

The standard display of coronary anatomy with conventional angiography includes views described by the position of the X-ray tube in relation to the patient. Standard views are, e.g. right anterior oblique (RAO 20), left anterior oblique (LAO 60), cranial, caudal, etc. VRIs allow visualization of the course of the coronary arteries in relation to the underlying cardiac chambers corresponding to the angiographic planes (**Figure 2.13**). Further evaluation is performed along individual segments or entire arteries using MPR and MIP. This can be achieved with manual reconstruction and semi-automated centreline reconstructions (**Figures 2.14** and **2.15**).

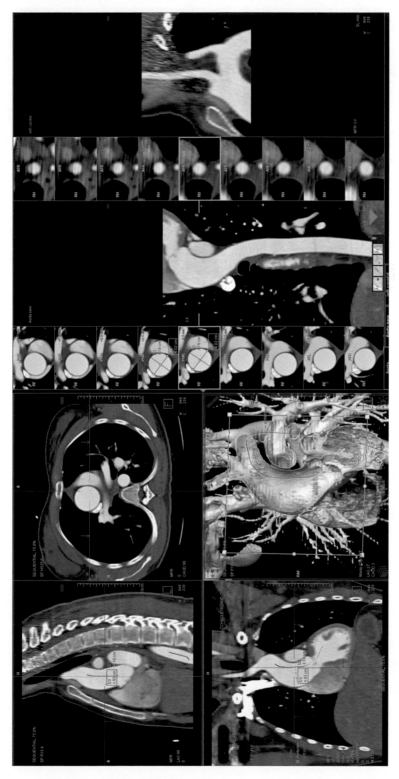

Figure 2.12 Aorta. The anatomy of the tubular aorta is reconstructed along the centreline of the vessel, with longitudinal and cross-sectional images. This can be done by manual reconstruction (left panels) or semi-automated centreline reconstructions (right panels). The origin of the arch branch vessels is identified.

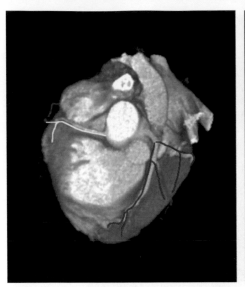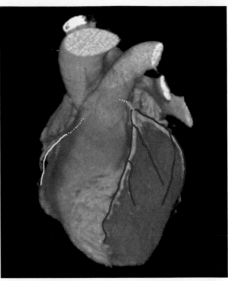

Figure 2.13 Coronary arteries, volume-rendered images (VRIs) of coronary arteries. This figure shows volume-rendered images (VRIs) of the heart corresponding to a LAO 60 view (right panel). Left main coronary artery (green), left anterior descending coronary artery (red), left circumflex coronary artery (blue), and right coronary artery (yellow). Volume-rendered images allow visualization of the course of the coronary arteries in relation to the underlying cardiac chambers corresponding to the angiographic planes.

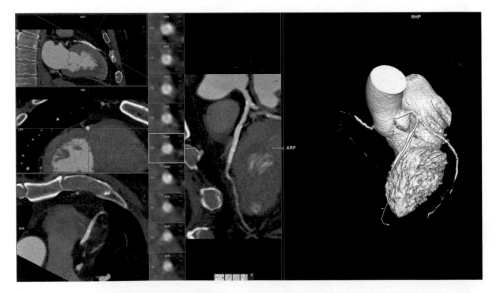

Figure 2.14 Segmental coronary visualization with CT. While volume-rendered images allow showing the course of the coronary arteries in relation underlying cardiac chambers corresponding to the angiographic planes, they do not allow detailed assessment of the complex coronary anatomy. This is achieved with dedicated coronary reconstruction along individual segments of the coronary arteries in multiple MPR and MIP images as shown in this figure. This figure shows a dedicated coronary reconstruction of the LAD with manual (left panels), semi-automated, centreline-based reconstructions (middle panel), and volume-rendered images (right panel).

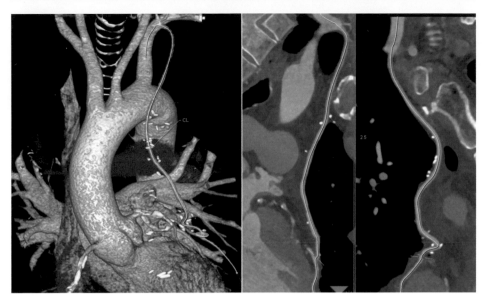

Figure 2.15 Centreline LIMA graft to LAD. This figure shows the centreline identified along the course of a LIMA graft to the LAD in VRI (left panel) and curved MPR images (two right panels)

2.1.3.6 Extracardiac structures: Lungs and mediastinum

The extracardiac structures are part of the CT acquisition volume and, in contrast to echocardiography and angiography, the acquired images are diagnostic. Therefore, careful review is part of CT analysis and reporting. A discussion of these structures is beyond the focus of this book. Modern software increasingly allows semi-automated, computer-aided analysis, specifically for lung nodule recognition.

Technical Aspects of Multidetector Computed Tomography

3.1 Data Acquisition

3.1.1 Current CT Systems

While current CT systems allow advanced cardiovascular imaging, important limitations remain, which are related to the following requirements of cardiovascular imaging:

1. High temporal resolution to avoid cardiac motion artefacts
2. High, isotropic (identical in-plane and through-plane) spatial resolution to visualize small anatomical details even on oblique reformats
3. Fast volume coverage during one breath-hold period to avoid respiratory motion artefacts
4. ECG synchronization of data acquisition or reconstruction to avoid cardiac motion artefacts

Scanners capable of ECG-synchronized scanning and 64 or more slices/rotation are now routinely used for cardiovascular imaging. Temporal resolution depends on the gantry rotation time (250–350 ms) and the number of X-ray sources (1 or 2). It ranges from 66 to 175 ms for scanners with 64 or more slices. These systems achieve an isotropic spatial resolution of $0.5 \times 0.5 \times 0.5$ mm^9 (**Figure 3.1**). The number of detector rows determines the volume covered in a single rotation. Most scanners cover between 20 and 160 mm per rotation. Coverage of the entire heart is possible with wide area detector scanners that permit 160 mm of coverage per rotation.

3.1.2 ECG Referencing

The rapid, constant motion of the heart causes significant image artefacts. The time between two consecutive heartbeats is described by the RR interval (the interval between consecutive R waves of the ECG, which is 1000 ms for a heart rate of 60 beats per minute [bpm]). Cardiac motion varies throughout the cardiac cycle, with minimal motion in diastole (about 75% RR-interval). A second window with limited motion is found in end systole (about 35% R-R interval). If motion-free images of the heart, aortic root, and ascending aorta are required, it is therefore important to synchronize data acquisition or reconstruction to the window with least cardiac motion. To avoid 'step artefacts' (**Figures 3.2** and **3.3**), synchronization of data is also a prerequisite to combine data acquired from consecutive gantry rotations in volumetric data sets.

Synchronization is based on observation of the ECG signal. The ECG signal is used to either prospectively trigger data acquisition or retrospectively gate data reconstruction to a certain

DOI: 10.1201/9781003153641-4

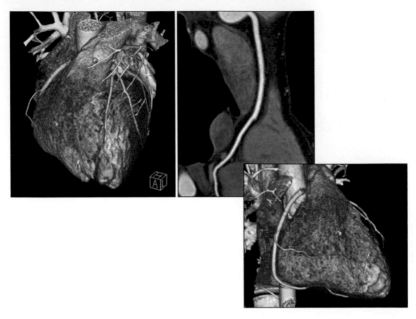

Figure 3.1 Current scanner systems. Modern CT systems with high spatial and temporal resolution allow imaging of the coronary arteries, which is particularly challenging, because of their small size, rapid motion, and tortuosity. This figure shows images of the coronary arteries acquired with a dual-source scanner with a temporal resolution of 75 ms. The volume-rendered images show the left and right coronary arteries. The curved MPR shows the LAD.

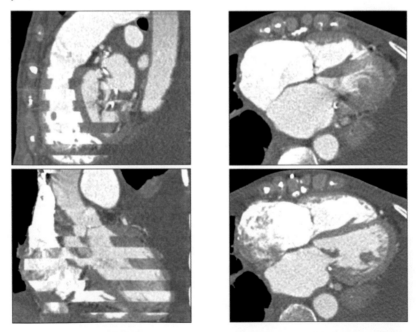

Figure 3.2 Arrhythmia artefact (1). A typical artefact can be seen in patients with arrhythmia and in particular atrial fibrillation. As shown in this figure, typical band-like shifts of the image data set are seen in image reconstructions. Each band represents the data obtained during one tube rotation and one heartbeat. Because the data acquisition is performed at slightly different phases in subsequent cardiac cycles, the reconstructed image stacks are misregistered.

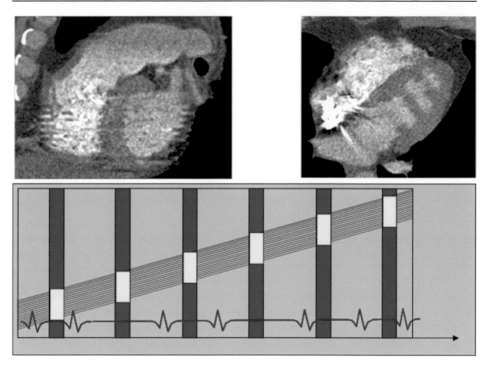

Figure 3.3 Arrhythmia artefact (2). Another example of a cardiac motion artefact is shown and illustrated in this figure. The typical band-like shifts of the image data set are more pronounced and thinner in these images from a prior generation four-detector row scanner.

phase of the cardiac cycle. The starting position of the data acquisition or reconstruction window is chosen in relation to the R wave of the ECG signal, typically using a relative delay value, which is defined as a given percentage of the RR interval.

For morphologic evaluation, data are usually selected from the diastolic phase of the cardiac cycle where heart motion is minimal, using a relative delay of 75% of the RR interval. However, the precise phase with minimal motion is patient-, scanner-, and heart rate–dependent, and should be optimized to ensure maximum image quality.[13,14] In addition, several reconstructions may be necessary, because different structures may reach minimal motion in slightly different phases of the cardiac cycle (e.g. left coronary artery [LCA] vs right coronary artery [RCA]). It is also important that data can be chosen from multiple phases throughout the cardiac cycle for functional evaluation.

3.1.3 Acquisition Mode

3.1.3.1 Sequential (axial) mode

Early CT systems (without slip ring) required the gantry to rewind to its initial position after each acquisition.[15] Individual transaxial image slices were acquired followed by incremental advancement of the patient table and repeated image acquisition at the next position (the 'stop and shoot' mode). Modern MDCT scanners can be operated in this sequential mode, but with continuous gantry rotation and acquisition of multiple slices per table position.

For these cardiovascular sequential protocols, data acquisition is prospectively triggered by the ECG signal, typically in late diastole. The main advantage of the sequential mode is lower radiation dose, because X-ray exposure occurs only during the prospectively triggered cardiac phase rather than throughout the entire cardiac cycle (X-ray source is turned on and off) and X-ray beam doesn't overlap as compared to the low-pitch spiral acquisition where the X-ray beam overlaps. Because image reconstruction is restricted to a single or a few phases of the cardiac cycle, this acquisition allows only limited correction in case of motion artefact. For these reasons, the prospective ECG-triggered sequential mode is reserved for patients with regular and low heart rates (typically < 60–65 bpm, but specific values depend on specific scanner characteristics and cardiovascular indication).[16] An additional limitation is that examination times are increased due to the need to increment the patient table between slice acquisitions except for wide area detector scanners with 160 mm of coverage per rotation.

3.1.3.2 Spiral (helical) mode

The initial development of multidetector row scanners for cardiovascular imaging was based on spiral data acquisition. In the spiral mode, data are acquired during constant rotation of the X-ray tube/detector system and continuous movement of the patient table through the gantry. For cardiac imaging, spiral data are retrospectively gated to the ECG signal. Data are acquired throughout the entire cardiac cycle, with simultaneous recording of the ECG signal. Data from specific periods of the cardiac cycle (most commonly late diastole) are then used for image reconstruction by retrospectively referencing to the ECG signal (retrospective ECG gating).[17] Because data are acquired throughout the cardiac cycle, spiral imaging allows reconstruction during multiple cardiac phases, which can be important for coronary imaging and is necessary for functional assessment. Retrospectively, ECG-gated spiral techniques are less sensitive to arrhythmia and allow faster volume coverage. Because X-ray exposure occurs throughout the cardiac cycle and X-ray beam overlaps, retrospective ECG-gated spiral techniques are generally associated with higher patient radiation doses, compared with imaging using sequential or non-synchronized techniques.

One scanner type, a dual-source CT scanner, capable of very fast spiral data acquisition using two X-ray tubes coupled with two detectors, allows scanning with a prospective ECG-triggered spiral acquisition mode. Spiral data acquisition is triggered by the patient's ECG signal to start during the diastolic phase and continues until the desired anatomic range is covered. The entire heart can be covered during a single diastolic phase for sufficiently low heart rates. Advantages of the prospective ECG-triggered spiral mode are lower radiation dose and extremely fast acquisition time. Like the prospective ECG-triggered sequential mode, this mode is sensitive to cardiac motion artefacts because of prospectively referencing to the ECG signal and is reserved for patients with low (<60 bpm) heart rates.[18]

3.1.4 Tube Current Modulation

The higher patient radiation dose with retrospectively ECG-gated spiral acquisition compared with prospectively ECG-triggered sequential or non-gated spiral techniques is in part the result of continuous X-ray exposure during the entire cardiac cycle. However, for most current cardiovascular clinical indications, only data from the diastolic phase are used for image

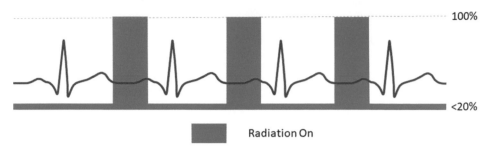

Figure 3.4 Minimal tube current outside the data acquisition window. This figure shows the reduction of the tube current by more than 80% outside the data acquisition window (diastolic phase) to decrease patient radiation exposure. Reconstruction of images in those low dose areas is still possible, but will have low image quality.

reconstruction. Modern scanners therefore allow reduction of the tube current by 80% or more outside the selected (diastolic) phase to decrease patient radiation exposure (**Figure 3.4**).[19] As a result, tube current and image quality are at a maximum only during the selected cardiac phase, but are reduced outside this phase. Therefore, while data are available during the entire cardiac cycle, image quality outside the selected (diastolic) phase is limited by increased noise (**Figure 3.5**). As a result, reconstruction at different phases, such as for optimizing coronary artery visualization or for functional analysis, is limited.

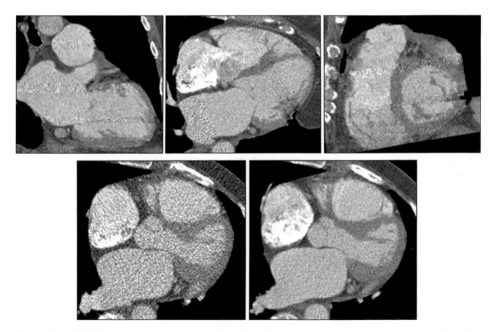

Figure 3.5 ECG-based tube current modulation. These are images of a patient in atrial fibrillation scanned with ECG-based tube current modulation. The oblique images in the upper row demonstrate bands of lower image quality, representing data acquisition outside the phase of maximum tube current. The difference in image quality (image noise) in axial images is demonstrated in the lower part of the figure.

3.1.5 Special Image Reconstruction Techniques to Improve Temporal Resolution

Modern CT scanners use several special imaging reconstruction techniques to improve temporal resolution. These include partial scan reconstructions and segmented reconstructions.

3.1.5.1 Partial scan reconstruction

Partial scan reconstruction algorithms reconstruct the individual axial image from data obtained during less than one complete rotation of the X-ray tube.[20] Because only approximately 180° of the projection data are needed for reconstruction, the temporal resolution for each axial image is reduced to one-half of the gantry rotation time. These reconstruction algorithms are used with sequential and spiral data and are the norm for cardiovascular CT reconstruction algorithms.

3.1.5.2 Multi-cycle reconstruction

Multi-cycle reconstruction algorithms can further improve temporal resolution.[21,22] Multi-cycle algorithms obtain the data used for reconstruction of an individual image from consecutive cardiac cycles. Therefore, the duration of the reconstruction window in each cycle can be reduced. These algorithms are particularly useful for patients with elevated heart rates, which are associated with significantly shorter diastolic windows of minimal motion.

Multi-cycle algorithms are implemented for retrospective ECG-gated spiral techniques on all single source CT scanners. These algorithms are also used for prospective ECG-triggered sequential scanning on a wide area detector system for patients with higher heart rates. The improvement in effective temporal resolution achieved with multi-cycle algorithms comes at a cost of increased radiation dose. Retrospectively, ECG-gated spiral techniques must be used with slower table movement (i.e., decreased pitch) resulting in higher radiation doses. For prospective ECG-triggered scans on a wide area detector system, the entire heart is imaged multiple times during repeated data acquisition (without table movement), thus increasing radiation dose. The number of heart cycles used for multi-cycle reconstruction is limited by several factors, and a maximum of two or three cycles is usually recommended for morphologic imaging. These algorithms typically result in effective temporal resolutions as low as 42–65 ms. It is important to note that the improvement in effective temporal resolution depends on the relationship between the gantry rotation time and the patient's heart rate, and optimal effective temporal resolution is achieved only for certain combinations of heart rate and gantry rotation time.

3.1.6 Radiation Exposure

The radiation exposure during a CT examination depends on the image protocol, which is dictated by the clinical question. Typical effective doses range between 1 and 10 mSv.

3.1.7 Contrast Media

Most cardiovascular CT protocols require the intravenous administration of iodinated contrast agents to enhance selected cardiovascular structures. Patients with renal insufficiency or contrast allergy are either pretreated (e.g. hydration, steroid treatment) or imaged with alternative modalities.

Standard contrast agents with an iodine concentration between 300 and 400 mg/mL are injected into an antecubital vein using power injectors, with typical injection rates of 3–5 mL/s. If peripheral access is not available, injection using central venous lines can be considered. Some of these are suitable for power injections, while others require hand injection. The amount of contrast agent required for a cardiac scan usually varies between 40 and 150 mL depending on the scan protocol and the scanner type.

Currently available contrast media are quickly diluted in the blood and distributed into the extracellular space, providing only a short time window for enhanced imaging. The transit time from the standard injection site (antecubital vein) to the heart is patient-dependent, and can vary between 20 and 40 s depending on the contrast flow rate and the patient's cardiac output. Therefore, determination of the scan delay (time between start of contrast agent injection and start of the scan) is critical to ensure optimal enhancement of the desired cardiovascular structures. This can be achieved with a small 'timing bolus' or by monitoring the diagnostic bolus ('bolus tracking'). With the use of a timing bolus, approximately 20 mL of contrast agent is injected, and a single image slice (typically at a level ~2 cm below the carina for imaging of the coronaries) is repeatedly imaged. The transit time of contrast agent to the region of interest (ROI) is determined from a time enhancement curve (**Figure 3.6**) and used for timing of the diagnostic bolus (**Figure 3.7**). Alternatively, with bolus tracking techniques, the entire diagnostic bolus is injected, and contrast enhancement is monitored in the ROI by repeated imaging at a single level. Once a certain enhancement threshold is achieved, breath-hold instructions are given, and scanning is started.

Bolus injection of contrast can lead to inhomogeneous enhancement, in particular in the superior vena cava (SVC) and right atrium (RA), where enhanced and non-enhanced

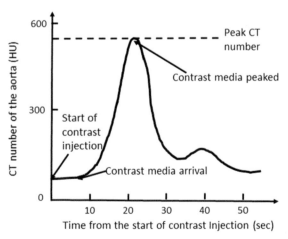

Figure 3.6 Time enhancement curve of ascending aorta. This is the time enhancement curve of the ascending aorta using the timing bolus technique. The time delay from the start of the bolus injection to the optimal contrast enhancement when the peak HU is reached is typically 20 to 40 s, depending on the injection rate and patient's cardiac output.

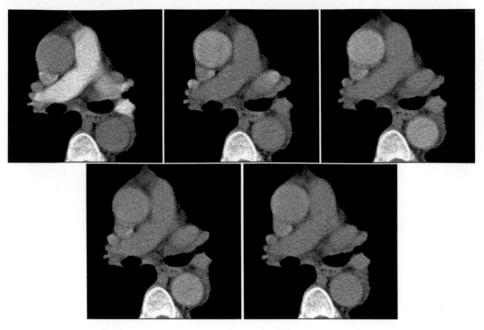

Figure 3.7 Test bolus. In this figure, enhancements of the ascending and descending aorta during the injection of a contrast bolus are shown. The left upper panel shows enhancement of the pulmonary artery, the right upper panel shows greater enhancement of the ascending than descending aorta and the lower left panel greater enhancement of the descending than ascending aorta.

blood meet (**Figure 3.8**). Non-uniform enhancement and the resulting beam-hardening artefacts may obscure right-sided structures, such as the pulmonary vessels and RCA. These artefacts in the SVC and RA may be reduced by scanning in the caudal–cranial direction, and by injection of a saline bolus following the contrast agent. Similarly, contrast injection at variable flow rates has been proposed to provide more prolonged, uniform enhancement of the aorta.[66,67]

3.1.7.1 Control of heart rate: Beta-blockers

Because of the association of lower heart rates with longer diastolic windows of minimal cardiac motion, cardiovascular CT image quality is improved for stable, slow heart rates. This is particularly important if small structures including the coronary arteries are examined. Although modern scanners allow correction for arrhythmia and higher heart rates (see the section 'Multi-Cycle Reconstruction'), heart rate control with oral or intravenous beta-blocker is routine for coronary CT angiography (CTA), if no contraindications exist (e.g. significant asthma, heart failure, aortic stenosis, heart block).[68,69] Alternatively, occasionally calcium-channel blockers are used.

3.1.7.2 Control of vessel tone: Nitroglycerin

Coronary CTA is typically performed after the sublingual administration of small nitroglycerin doses for vessel dilatation. The rationale is that visualization of a dilated vessel is improved.

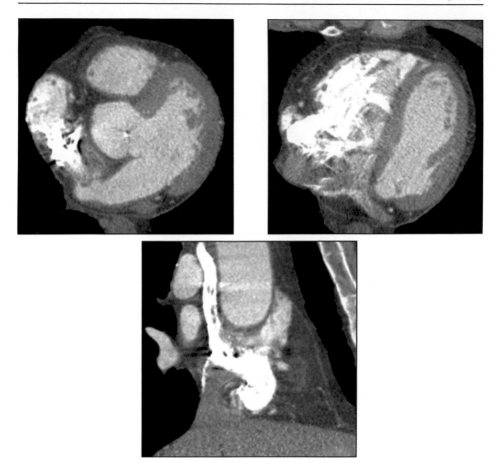

Figure 3.8 Streak artefact/contrast material. Bolus injection of contrast can lead to inhomogeneous enhancement in particular of the superior vena cava (SVC) and right atrium (RA), where enhanced and non-enhanced blood mixes. This figure shows axial images at the interface between the SVC and RA (left upper) and inferior VC and RA (right upper) and a sagittal reconstruction (lower panel). Non-uniform enhancement and the resulting beam-hardening artefacts may obscure right-sided structures, such as the pulmonary vessels and right coronary artery.

3.1.8 Energy Integrating Detector (EID) and Photon Counting Detector (PCD) CT

As mentioned in the beginning of this chapter, one of the limitations of current CT scanners is insufficient spatial resolution. CT is an excellent diagnostic tool to rule out coronary artery disease in relatively large vessels, but due to limited spatial resolution which also causes 'blooming' from calcified plaques, its assessment of coronary artery stenosis is less reliable. Due to the same limitation, the evaluation of stent patency and in-stent re-stenosis is mostly reliable for stents with a diameter no less than 3 mm.

Photon counting CT uses a new type of detector material – cadmium telluride (CdTe) or cadmium zinc telluride (CZT)[23] – which can convert individual X-ray photon directly into a cloud of charges of electron-hole pairs (**Figure 3.9**), as compared to conventional

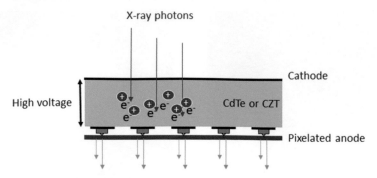

Figure 3.9 Photon counting detector. In a Photon Counting Detector, X-ray photons interact directly with semiconductor material, such as CdTe or CZT, to create electron-hole pairs. Under strong electric field between cathode and pixelated anodes, electrons drift to the anodes and induce current pulses, which last a few nanoseconds. Since the strong electrical field defines the detector cell boundary, there is no need to have highly reflecting septa between detector cells.

solid-state scintillation detectors, which generate signals in two steps: (1) the scintillation crystal converts absorbed X-ray photons into visible light photons, and (2) visible light photons are converted into electrons by photodiodes attached to the back of the detector cell (**Figure 3.10**), and then integrated into detector signals. Because of the integration step, conventional CT detector is also called 'energy integrating detector' (EID). The final signal from EID detector is the contribution from all X-ray photons during the signal readout, and information about the energy of each individual photon is lost. As a contrary, each individual X-ray photon will be counted in PCD if the charge-induced pulse exceeds certain limit, which is typically set to be high enough to exclude the electrical noises. Unlike conventional EID detector, PCD doesn't need highly reflecting septa between detector cells because individual detector cell is defined by the strong electric field between the cathode and pixelated anodes; therefore, the detector cell can be further divided into smaller detector sub-cells without sacrificing dose efficiency. One commercially available photon counting CT Naeotom Alpha (Siemens Healthineers, Erlangen, Germany) can divide detector cell (0.5×0.5 mm^2) into four sub-cells (0.225×0.225 mm^2) for the ultrahigh resolution (UHR) mode.

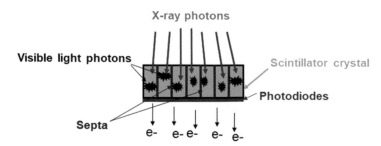

Figure 3.10 Conventional energy integrating detector. In a conventional Energy Integrating Detector, incident X-ray photons interact with the scintillation crystals to convert their energy into visible light photons. The light photons are absorbed by photodiodes and converted into electrons, which are integrated into electrical current. (To prevent optical crosstalk, highly reflecting septa are used to separate the detector cells.)

The other benefits of photon counting CT come from its ability to differentiate X-ray photons based on their energies. The energy resolved (with multiple energy levels, not just dual energy) CT data is important for material decomposition which can provide quantitative information of soft tissue (water), iodine contrast, calcium (bone), or other contrast media (k-edge imaging). In photon counting CT, low energy X-ray photon is counted the same as the high-energy photon, as compared to the conventional EID detector, in which high energy X-ray photon is weighted more in the integrated signal due to its ability to generate more visible light photons. As a result, photon counting CT can significantly improve the image contrast, especially in CT scans with iodinated contrast agent, since the image contrast is mainly contributed by the low energy X-ray photons.

3.1.9 Imaging Protocols

A critical step in obtaining clinically meaningful results is careful planning of the CT examination protocols according to the specific clinical indication. The first step in protocol planning is to decide whether prospectively triggered sequential (axial) or fast spiral acquisition mode (only available on dual-source CT) can be used. These scan modes typically offer the lowest radiation dose to the patient, but only applicable to the patients with regular and low heart rates. For patients with high heart rate or arrhythmia, or those requiring functional assessment, a retrospective ECG-gated spiral mode is a better choice. Once the scan mode is decided, selection of the tube voltage (kVp) can be the next step. Low kVp (100 kVp or lower) is associated with lower radiation dose and brighter iodine contrast, but only works for regular to small size patient. Some CT scanners offer automatic kVp selection feature, i.e., the scanner can select optimal kVp based on the patient attenuation estimate from the scout scan. If the scanner doesn't offer this feature, a manual chart for kVp selection based on the patient size (BMI, chest dimension, etc.) is also helpful. The selection of the reconstruction kernels can have huge impact on the spatial resolution and noise. High spatial resolution reconstruction kernels are usually reserved for visualization of small cardiac anatomy (e.g. coronary arteries) or stent, but it comes with the penalty of elevated image noise. In conventional CT reconstruction (filtered back projection, or FBP), the spatial resolution and image noise are always a trade-off. A more advanced reconstruction algorithm developed over the past few years is the iterative reconstruction, which can be used to reduce the image noise while still maintaining the spatial resolution of most high-contrast objects, such as stent or calcified plaque. For imaging relatively large cardiac anatomy, such as the aorta, the spatial resolution may not be as critical. In that case, thicker slice thickness or smooth reconstruction kernel can be used to reduce the image noise, and therefore lower the radiation dose.

For protocols used for quantitative assessment of calcium or iodine, such as calcium scoring protocol, the selection of reconstruction kernel is critical, because some kernels may have edge enhancement or other image manipulation features, which may impact the accuracy of Hounsfield unit (HU) values. It is important to consult with CT vendors on the selection of the reconstruction kernel for those applications requiring accurate measurement of the attenuation from calcium or iodine contrast.

3.1.10 Image Artefacts

The recognition of image artefacts is important in order to avoid false-positive diagnosis. Artefacts are often related to patient characteristics, the quality control, and technical limitations of CT.

3.1.10.1 Cardiac motion artefact

Because of the rapid motion of the heart and the relatively long acquisition window, blurring of the image occurs, in particular if the acquisition window is not synchronized to the cardiac cycle. An important example is motion artefact at the root of the aorta in non–ECG-gated studies (**Figure 3.11**). This artefact becomes more significant if smaller structures, including the coronary arteries, are imaged (**Figure 3.12**).

3.1.10.2 Arrhythmia artefact

A typical motion artefact can be seen in patients with arrhythmia, particularly atrial fibrillation. As shown in **Figures 3.2** and **3.3**, typical band-like shifts of the image data are seen in image reconstructions. Each band represents the data obtained during one tube rotation and one heartbeat. Because of the irregular heart rate, data acquisition occurs at

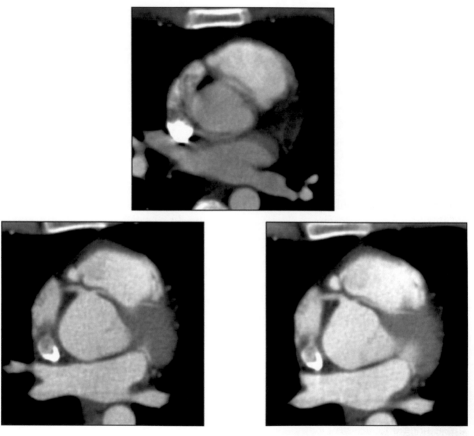

Figure 3.11 Motion artefact: Anomalous coronary artery. In this figure, images of a mildly dilated aortic root are shown at the level of the RCA origin. The upper panel shows non–ECG-gated images. Motion artefact precludes precise assessment of coronary artery anatomy. The patient had repeated imaging 2 years later and an ECG-referenced protocol was performed (lower panels). These images show the anomalous origin of the left main from the right coronary cusp adjacent to the RCA ostium.

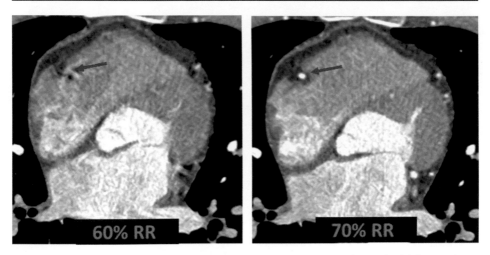

Figure 3.12 Motion artefact: Image reconstruction window. In this figure, the left image shows completely blurred RCA reconstructed using 60% RR interval. By changing the reconstruction window to 70% RR interval, the RCA is no longer blurred in the image on the right.

slightly different phases in subsequent cardiac cycles. Changes in ventricular size during systole and diastole can, therefore, lead to misregistration of images. Similar artefacts occur in patients with extrasystolic beats (**Figures 3.13** and **3.14**). Most modern CT systems allow editing of the detected R peaks of the ECG signal.

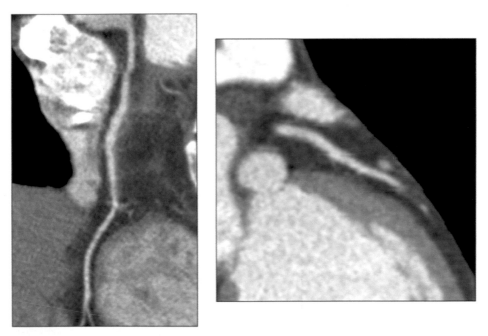

Figure 3.13 Arrhythmia artefact: Extrasystole (1). An example of misregistration secondary to an extrasystole is shown in this image. Modern scanners allow limited editing of these artefacts, e.g. by deleting the information of a single irregular beat, often with significant improvement of image quality.

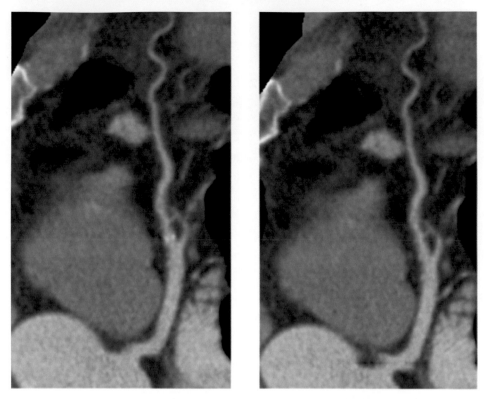

Figure 3.14 Arrhythmia artefact: Extrasystole (2). The images in this figure show other examples of arrhythmia artefact. There is misregistration in the proximal left main coronary artery.

3.1.10.3 Partial volume averaging

Small structures with high CT numbers (HU), e.g. calcium or metallic material (coronary stents, surgical clips), cause a characteristic artefact, which often precludes assessment of adjacent structures. This partial volume averaging artefact (or blooming artefact) arises because an object with a high CT number, which is smaller than the voxel size, increases the CT number of the entire voxel, represented on the CT image. Therefore, the object size is overestimated. The partial volume averaging artefact can be reduced by reconstructing images with thinner slice thickness (**Figure 3.15**). To reduce the blooming related to the highly attenuating object, increasing the tube voltage is also helpful.

3.1.10.4 Beam hardening artefacts

Beam hardening artefacts are caused by preferential attenuation of low energy X-ray photons by patient. For X-ray photons generated by a CT tube, there is a distribution of X-ray photon energies, ranging from a few keVs all the way to the peak voltage (e.g. 120 keV for the 120 kVp X-ray beam). Due to preferential attenuation of low energy X-ray photons, there are more high energy X-ray photons left in the beam after the beam passes through the attenuating object, such as a water cylinder (**Figure 3.16**), hence the X-ray beam is 'hardened.' The effect of 'hardened' X-ray beam received by the CT detector causes incorrect measurement of the attenuation, especially for those highly attenuating objects (e.g. iodine contrast, metallic

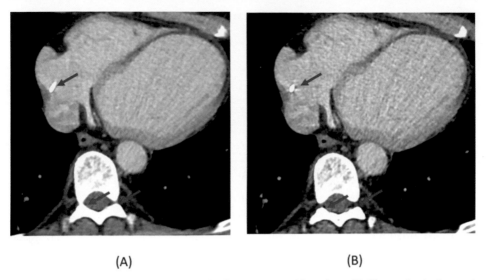

(A)   (B)

Figure 3.15 Partial volume artefacts: Iodine contrast blooming. (A) Shows the iodine and calcium blooming (red arrows) due to partial volume averaging in thicker slice (3 mm). (B) this image is reconstructed with a thinner slice (1 mm) for the same CT scan on the left. The iodine and calcium blooming is significantly reduced for the thinner slice images due to decreased partial volume averaging.

implant) or anatomical structures (e.g. bones). **Figure 3.17** shows typical beam hardening artefacts caused by iodine contrast.

3.1.10.5 Streak artefact: Metallic implants

Large areas of high-density material, in particular metallic foreign bodies, can severely reduce X-ray transmission. In the extreme, the detector may not record any signal transmission,

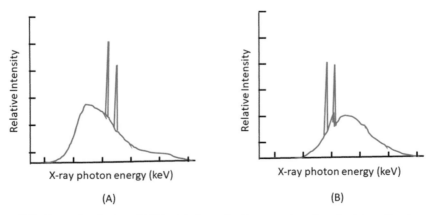

(A)   (B)

Figure 3.16 Beam hardening. (A) This plot shows the X-ray spectrum from the tube without passing through any attenuating material. (B) This plot shows the X-ray spectrum after attenuated by 20 cm water. The low-energy photons were absorbed by water more than the high-energy photons; therefore, the mean energy of the beam is higher on the right, or it is considered being 'hardened' by the attenuating material, which is water in this case.

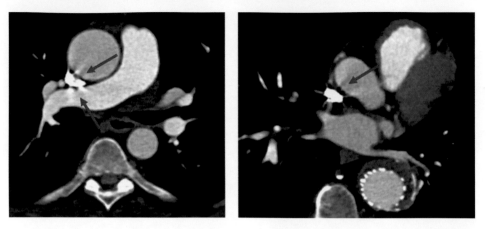

Figure 3.17 Beam hardening artefacts from iodine contrast. Like other highly attenuating materials, iodine contrast can cause severe beam hardening artefacts when the iodine concentration is high and low kVp technique is used. In these two images, the iodine contrast caused severe shading bands (red arrow) on the adjacent anatomies.

causing the reconstruction algorithm to fail, and produce streaks in the image originating from the source object. This has implications for cardiovascular imaging, as metal implants are common. Examples are pacer/implantable cardioverter defibrillator (ICD) wires, endovascular stents, and surgical material (**Figure 3.18**).

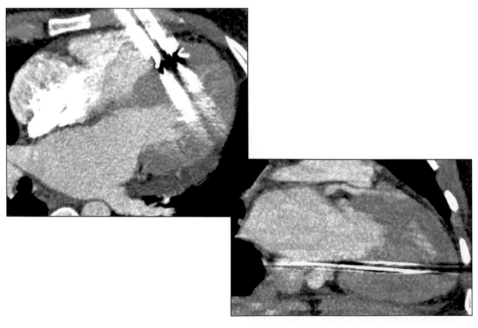

Figure 3.18 Streak artefact/metallic implants. The metal lead of pacer/ICD wires causes a strong artefact, which often precludes precise assessment of position as shown in these images.

3.1.10.6 Streak artefact: Contrast material

Similar streak artefact is also caused by iodinated contrast. Particularly in the SVC and RA, high-iodine concentration contrast material and areas of mixing between contrast-rich and unenhanced blood can cause significant artefact, often precluding assessment of adjacent structures (**Figure 3.8**).

Most CT vendors offer metal artefacts reduction (MAR) feature to reduce the streak artefacts caused by the metal implant, and in some degree, the streaks caused by the iodinated contrast. However, due to the empirical nature of most MAR techniques, the degree of artefacts reduction varies, and depends on the size, shape, and material composition of the metallic object.

Section 2

Clinical Cardiovascular Applications

4

Cardiac Chambers and Myocardial Disease

Imaging is an essential part in the diagnostic work-up of patients with cardiovascular disease. Multiple imaging modalities are established and utilization has increased significantly. However, invasive and non-invasive imaging is associated with a small risk of complications and significant cost. Therefore, in clinical practice, a presumptive diagnosis is initially formed based on physical examination and history, and the most appropriate imaging modality is then chosen to confirm or refute this diagnosis. This focused approach requires knowledge about strength and limitations of the individual imaging modalities for specific clinical scenarios, but is best suited to ensure appropriate use of imaging resources. Systematic textbooks of cardiovascular medicine[24] describe the clinical perspective, while consensus guidelines discuss appropriate indications.[25-27]

The following clinical chapters of the manual are not intended to provide a comprehensive description of cardiovascular imaging, but are in introduction to the role of MDCT for common clinical cardiovascular indications.

4.1 Cardiac Chambers and Myocardium

Contrast-enhanced CT provides detailed anatomic information about the cardiac chambers and the myocardium. It is primarily a static anatomic modality, which is utilized if morphologic findings are in question. The high spatial resolution and ability to reconstruct the acquired 3-D data set along oblique axes allow assessment of global and focal myocardial pathology. CT can therefore provide useful information in patients with non-ischemic and ischemic cardiomyopathies. However, in the assessment of these conditions the evaluation of ventricular function and integrity of the valvular structures is essential, and therefore echocardiography and magnetic resonance imaging (MRI) are typically the initial tests of choice. CT data acquisition throughout the cardiac cycle (retrospective gating) and subsequent reconstructions along different phases of the cardiac cycle put together into cine loops allow for limited functional assessment. However, because of lower temporal resolution, associated contrast and radiation exposure, its role is typically restricted to clinical scenarios in which echocardiography and MRI are not possible or significantly limited. In the assessment of left ventricular (LV) measurements with MDCT, studies show a good correlation of left ventricular ejection fraction (LVEF) values with cine-MRI, but significant under-estimation of LV volumes with MDCT.

DOI: 10.1201/9781003153641-6

4.2 Cardiomyopathies

4.2.1 Non-Ischemic Cardiomyopathies

4.2.1.1 Dilated cardiomyopathy (DCM)

The typical findings in patients with DCM are ventricular dilatation with diffuse, relative thinning of the myocardium (**Figure 4.1**).[28] These findings can involve the left and right ventricle (RV) and are associated with various degrees of ventricular dysfunction.

In contrast to patients with ischemic cardiomyopathy, the coronary arteries are typically normal or only mildly diseased. In the initial clinical assessment of patients with suspected non-ischemic cardiomyopathy, an assessment of coronary anatomy is typically performed, either with conventional angiography or non-invasive CT angiography.[29]

4.2.1.2 Left ventricular non-compaction phenotype (LVNC)

Left-ventricular non-compaction describes excessive and prominent trabeculations associated with deep recesses that communicate with the ventricular cavity (**Figures 4.2–4.4**).[30] Prominent trabeculations are a normal feature of the developing myocardium *in utero*

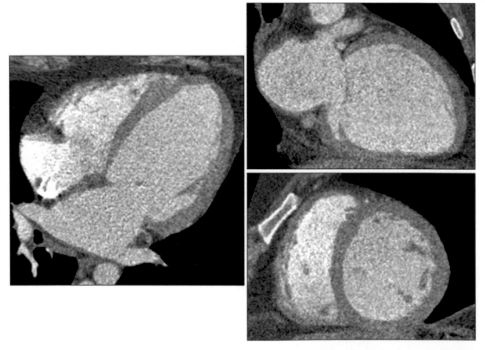

Figure 4.1 Dilated cardiomyopathy. This figure shows end-diastolic images of a patient with non-ischemic cardiomyopathy. There is moderate-to-severe left ventricular dilatation, thinning of the myocardial wall, but no evidence of focal scarring. The right ventricle is normal in size. There is no evidence of thrombus within the cardiac chambers. There was no evidence of coronary artery disease.

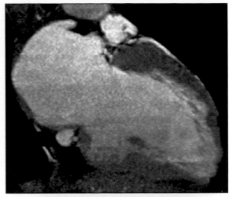

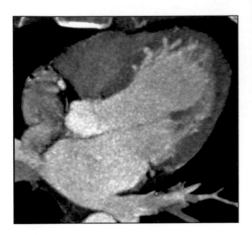

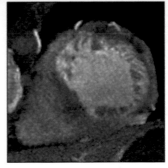

Figure 4.2 Left ventricular non-compaction (CT). A young patient presented with fatigue and palpitations. An exercise stress echocardiogram demonstrated deep horizontal inferior ST depression and a significant decrease in ejection fraction. CT demonstrates pronounced trabeculations of the anterior and inferior wall, consistent with left ventricular non-compaction.

and LVNC is thought to result from a failure of trabecular regression that occurs during normal embryonic development. Because the development extends from basal septum to the apical lateral wall, there is often a transition point between compacted and non-compacted myocardium.

The diagnosis of LVNC is usually made using echocardiography and MRI, but there are conflicting definitions of LVNC.[31-34] Some criteria require a double-layered appearance of the myocardium on 2-D echocardiography and cardiac magnetic resonance (CMR) imaging and others require only prominent or numerous LV trabeculations. While LVNC was originally considered as a distinct entity, more recent data describes non-compaction as a phenotype associated with different cardiomyopathies.[35-37]

4.2.1.3 Hypertrophic cardiomyopathy (HCM) and hypertrophic obstructive cardiomyopathy (HOCM)

This group of cardiomyopathies is characterized by primary myocardial hypertrophy.[38] Different entities have characteristic distributions of the hypertrophic myocardium. Apical HCM (Yamaguchi) is characterized by concentric LV thickening in the distal and apical LV segments (**Figures 4.5** and **4.6**). The classic morphologic finding in patients with HOCM is

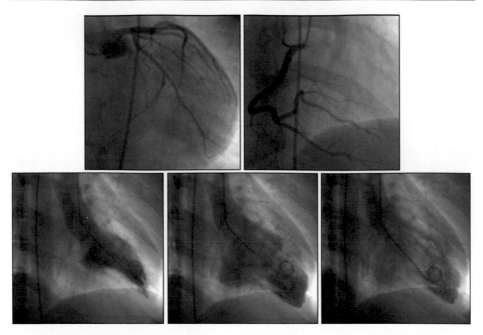

Figure 4.3 Left ventricular non-compaction (angiography) (1). The corresponding angiographic images confirm the areas of trabeculation. There was no evidence of stenotic disease of the epicardial coronary arteries. Cardiac MRI with delayed contrast-enhanced imaging showed no evidence of myocardial scar.

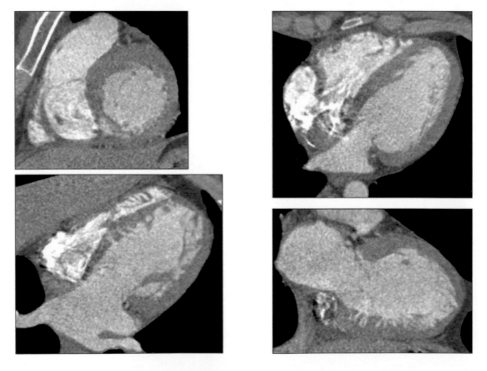

Figure 4.4 Left ventricular non-compaction (2). In this figure, prominent trabeculations are obvious in the inferior and lateral wall of the left ventricle.

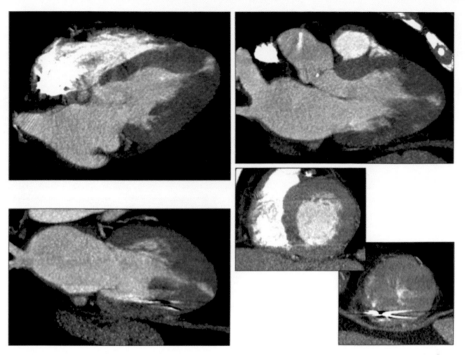

Figure 4.5 Apical hypertrophic cardiomyopathy (1). The typical distribution of apical hypertrophy (Yamaguchi) is shown in this figure. Systolic contraction leads to obstruction of the distal left ventricular cavity. The wire of a defibrillator system (ICD) is seen ending in the right ventricle.

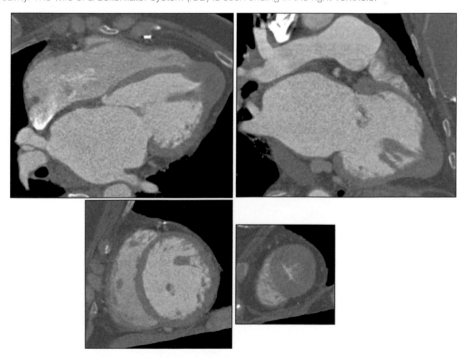

Figure 4.6 Apical hypertrophic cardiomyopathy (2). Focal apical hypertrophy limited to the left ventricular apex is shown in this image.

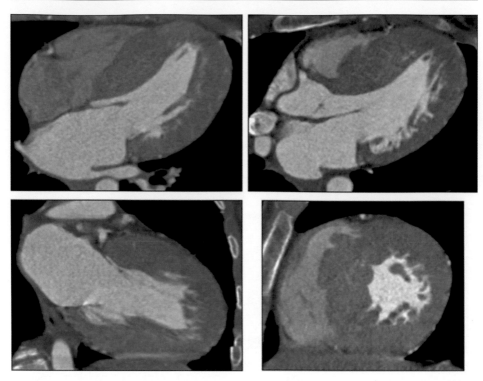

Figure 4.7 Hypertrophic obstructive cardiomyopathy (HOCM) (a). The morphologic findings of HOCM are demonstrated in the following figures. In this figure, diffuse hypertrophy of the left ventricle with an asymmetric thickening (3 cm) involving the basal interventricular septum is shown.

asymmetric septal hypertrophy (**Figures 4.7–4.10**). However, functional evidence of outflow tract obstruction during rest and stress (typically assessed with echocardiography) is necessary for the diagnosis. Non-obstructive HCM is differentiated by the absence of outflow tract obstruction.

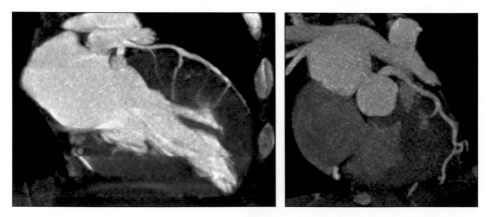

Figure 4.8 HOCM (b). This figure shows normal coronary anatomy of the left anterior descending (LAD) artery. Treatment consists of either partial surgical resection of the septal myocardium or percutaneous ablation using selective alcohol injection into septal branches of the LAD. The location of the septal branches is visible.

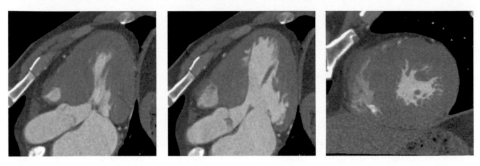

Figure 4.9 HOCM (c). In this patient, the three-chamber view shows partial obstruction of the left ventricular outflow tract by the hypertrophic basal interventricular septum. Besides, the systolic and diastolic images show systolic anterior motion of the anterior mitral leaflet (SAM). The short axial image shows severe basal septum hypertrophy.

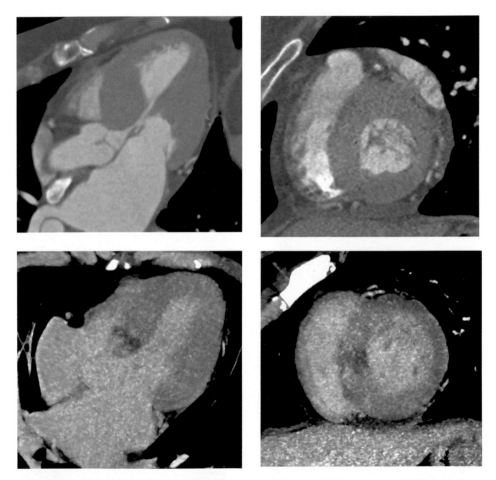

Figure 4.10 HOCM with pre- and post-therapy. A 51-year-old female with HOCM underwent alcohol septal myocardial ablation. The upper panel shows the pre-ablation MDCT images, with obstruction of the left ventricular outflow tract and thickened myocardium of the interventricular septum. Ten months after septal ablation, there is no residual obstruction in the LV outflow tract (lower panels). There is a low-density lesion in the basal septum myocardium, suggested necrosis in this area.

Assessment of scar is typically performed with MRI (gadolinium-delayed imaging) but has recently been described with CT.[39,40]

4.2.1.4 Restrictive cardiomyopathy (RCM)

Restrictive cardiomyopathies describe a group of disease conditions that are characterized by increased ventricular stiffness. A diagnostic hallmark is diastolic dysfunction, which is best assessed with echocardiography. Ventricular stiffness can be secondary to myocardial infiltration (e.g. cardiac amyloidosis), where advanced disease stages potentially show myocardial prominence and can involve both LV and RV wall (**Figures 4.11** and **4.12**).[41] Restriction can also be caused by endocardial fibrosis (e.g. Loeffler's endocarditis) (**Figure 4.13**).

4.2.1.5 Arrhythmogenic right ventricular dysplasia (ARVD)

Arrhythmogenic right ventricular dysplasia describes a clinical syndrome of life-threatening ventricular tachycardia, originating from foci of a remodelled RV wall.[42] Major and minor diagnostic criteria have been described.[43] Major imaging criteria are severe RV dilatation with regional RV dysfunction, and localized RV aneurysms (**Figure 4.14**). Minor criteria

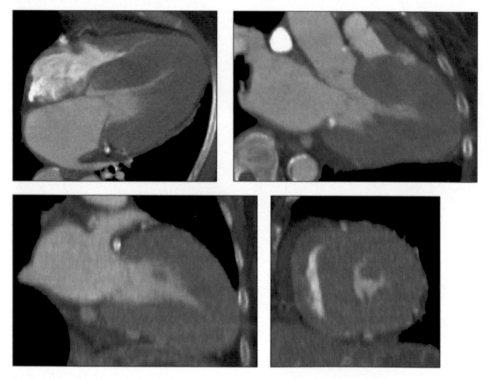

Figure 4.11 Cardiac amyloidosis (1). This figure shows severe, diffuse, left- and right-sided wall thickening with overall diffuse enlargement of the left and right ventricle. This appearance is unusual for left ventricular hypertrophy secondary to hypertensive heart disease and is consistent with an infiltrative processes including amyloidosis, or hypertrophic cardiomyopathy.

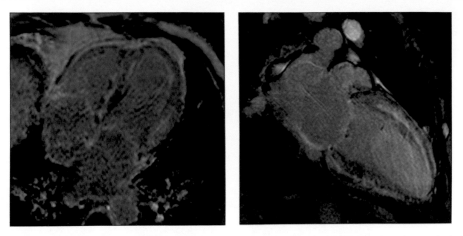

Figure 4.12 Cardiac amyloidosis (2). Delayed contrast-enhanced MRI imaging demonstrated characteristic patterns of fibrosis in patients with cardiac amyloidosis. As shown in this figure, typically a global and subendocardial pattern of enhancement is observed.

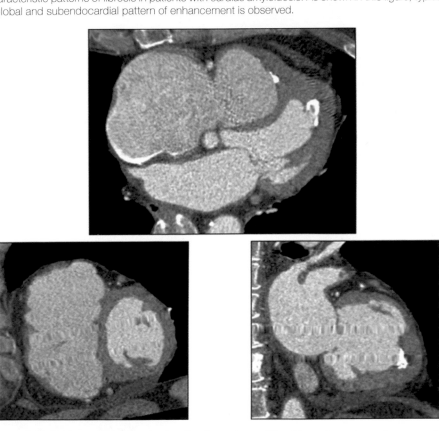

Figure 4.13 Endocardial fibrosis, Loeffler's endocarditis. These images are from a patient with endocardial fibrosis secondary to Loefflers's endocarditis. There is severe enlargement of the right atrium and moderately severe enlargement of the right ventricle with a reversal of normal interventricular septal curvature. There are bulky areas of calcification in the myocardium of the right and left ventricular apices, with blunting of the ventricular cavities and deformity in the configuration both ventricles due to apical scar tissue combined with dense calcification. The calcification in the right atrium is most consistent with a layered, calcified thrombus.

47

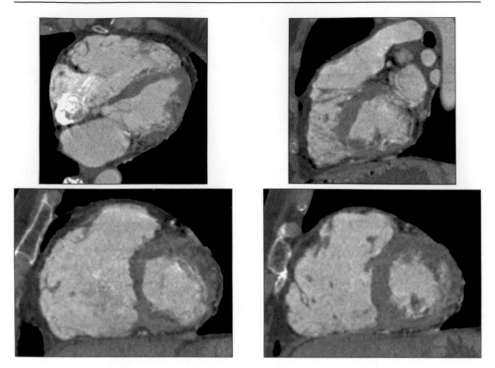

Figure 4.14 Arrhythmogenic right ventricular dysplasia (ARVD). The images in this figure demonstrate severe dilatation of the right ventricle. Further evaluation of the right ventricular wall is notable for small aneurysms of the wall. Together these abnormalities are supportive of the diagnosis of ARVD.

are mild RV dilatation and/or reduced ejection fraction, mild segmental dilatation, and regional RV hypokinesia.

The major and minor criteria are defined for echocardiography and MRI.[43] Both modalities have high diagnostic accuracy for major and minor criteria, because of their reliable visualization of RV anatomy and function. While dynamic reconstruction of spiral CT data allows visualization of RV wall motion, CT has limited temporal resolution and no significant role in functional assessment. Its use is limited to selected patients with poor echocardiographic images and contraindications to MRI (e.g. presence of defibrillator).

MRI and CT allow characterizing myocardial wall abnormalities including thinning, and focal aneurysm formation. The identification of focal fibrous or fatty replacement of myocardium involving the RV and sometimes LV myocardium is sometimes possible with MRI or CT. However, these finding are difficult to identify and non-specific and are not included in current guidelines.

4.2.2 Ischemic Cardiomyopathy

4.2.2.1 Acute coronary syndromes

The clinical imaging approach to patients presenting with suspected high likelihood of an acute coronary syndrome is based on the emergent, early assessment of coronary anatomy in order to identify potential 'target/culprit lesions' for subsequent revascularization. Because of its reliable definition of highly stenotic lesions and the ability for immediate therapeutic intervention, conventional angiography remains the test of choice for assessment of coronary anatomy in the acute setting. In addition, bedside assessment of LV wall motion abnormalities and ejection fraction is critical and typically performed with echocardiography.

Clinical observations describe areas of decreased contrast enhancement in hypoperfused myocardial segments with MRI and CT (**Figures 4.15** and **4.16**).[44] However, in the acute phase, MRI and CT are of limited use, mainly because of the long acquisition time and limited ability for critical monitoring for MRI and additional contrast administration for CT. The role of these modalities is however evaluated in the subacute phase:

- MRI data describes comprehensive evaluation of patients with acute myocardial infarction after primary revascularization. In these patients, MRI 'edema' and 'scar' imaging allow to define irreversible damage and areas of potential resolution ('salvage index').[45–48] Cardiac CT in patients after primary PCI without additional contrast has demonstrated areas of retained myocardial contrast.[49,50]
- In patient presenting to the ED with chest pain but intermediate suspicion and initial negative ECG and cardiac enzymes, the role of CT for early triage has been examined in several large multicentre trials.[51–54] However, these results need to be evaluated in the context of other test, specifically hs-troponin.[55]

CT and MRI also have an established role in the evaluation of subacute complications of acute myocardial infarction, including free wall rupture and pseudoaneurysm formation (**Figures 4.17** and **4.18**).[56]

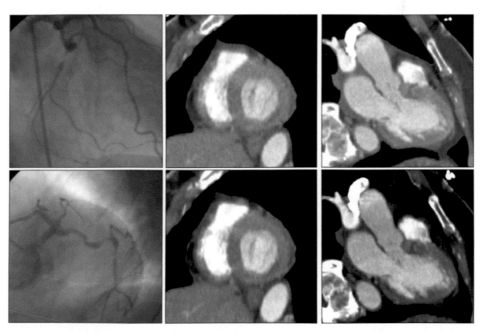

Figure 4.15 Myocardial perfusion defect. This figure shows an example of a myocardial perfusion defect of the inferior-posterior and septal wall. The posterolateral and inferoseptal regions demonstrate decreased subendocardial contrast enhancement consistent with hypoperfusion. This area is better seen on the MIP images (lower panel). On the angiogram, there is diffused severely stenotic atherosclerotic disease of the left circumflex and left anterior descending coronary arteries.

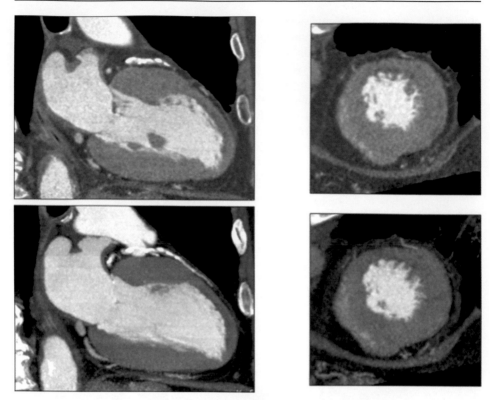

Figure 4.16 Chronic myocardial perfusion defect. This figure shows an example of a chronic perfusion defect of the anterior wall. The patient had a remote history of myocardial infarction and had a CT performed to define aortic anatomy. The cardiac chambers are notable for mild left ventricular hypertrophy except for the mid to apical anterior wall, corresponding to the LAD distribution, which shows myocardial thinning, consistent with previous myocardial infarction. There is a small area of decreased subendocardial contrast enhancement consistent with hypoperfusion. This area is better seen on the MIP images (lower panel). Corresponding to the area of previous infarction, the LAD has diffused atherosclerotic changes with densely calcified lesions.

4.2.2.2 Chronic ischemic cardiomyopathy

Areas of remote LV myocardial infarction typically demonstrate ventricular wall thinning with fibrous or calcified replacement of myocardium, and aneurysm formation with or without cavitary thrombus (**Figures 4.19–4.23**).[56] Focal aneurysms can be differentiated from diverticula by the lack of contraction on functional studies.

4.3 Other Cardiac and Myocardial Conditions

4.3.1 Myocarditis

Myocarditis is associated with acute chest pain and elevated troponin and can lead to DCM. Clinical presentations, biochemistry, and echocardiographic findings may overlap with those of myocardial infarction or ischemic heart disease. Imaging plays a central role in the diagnosis. Echocardiography and CMR are established non-invasive imaging modalities

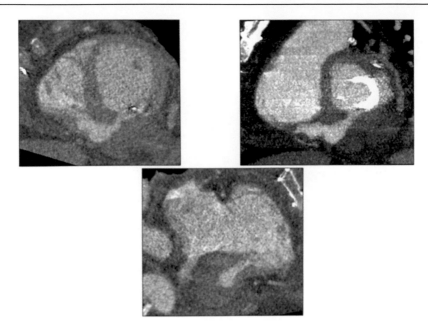

Figure 4.17 Contained LV rupture and pseudoaneurysm. This figure shows short-axis (upper panels) and two-chamber (lower panel) images from a patient with an infero-basal left ventricular pseudoaneurysm after acute myocardial infarction. A partially contrast-filled pseudoaneurysm originates from the inferior aspect of the left ventricle and extends under both ventricles. There is evidence of mitral valve replacement with a bioprosthetic valve.

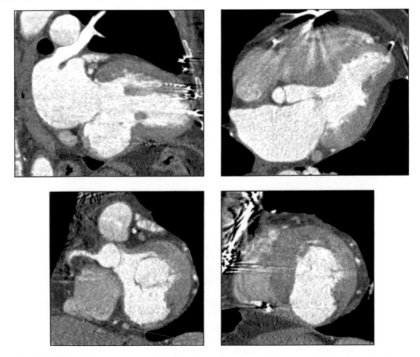

Figure 4.18 LV Pseudoaneurysm. This figure shows images from a patient with an infero-basal left ventricular pseudoaneurysm after an acute myocardial infarction. A contrast-filled pseudoaneurysm originates from the basal inferior aspect of the left ventricle and extends under the mitral valve.

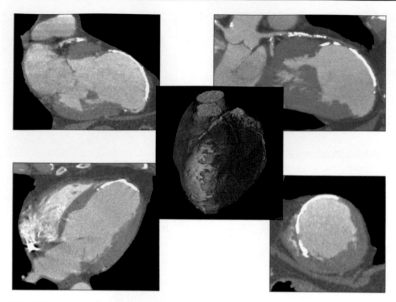

Figure 4.19 Calcified left ventricular aneurysm. This figure shows images of a patient with coronary artery disease. There is dense calcified disease of the proximal to mid-LAD, with a post-infarct aneurysm of the anterior left ventricular myocardium. There is overall moderate left ventricular dilatation. Beginning at the junction of the proximal and middle thirds of the left ventricle, there is pronounced myocardial thinning including the anterior and septal segments with relative sparing of the anterolateral and lateral regions. The area of thinning demonstrates bulging compatible with true aneurysm formation extending to the apex. The infarcted wall is densely calcified without evidence of adherent mural thrombus.

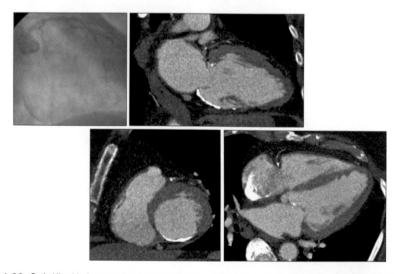

Figure 4.20 Calcified left ventricular aneurysm. This figure shows images of a patient with known coronary artery disease. During a cardiac catheterization an area of calcification in the inferior basal segment of the left ventricle was noted and pericardial calcification was suspected (left upper panel). However, the subsequent CT demonstrated myocardial calcification consistent with myocardial scar. The left ventricle is notable for myocardial thinning of the basal and mid-inferior wall. There is associated calcification of the base of the inferior wall beginning at the level of the mitral annulus. The pericardium has normal thickness without any evidence of calcification. There is severe calcification of all three coronary arteries. These findings are consistent with remote myocardial infarction.

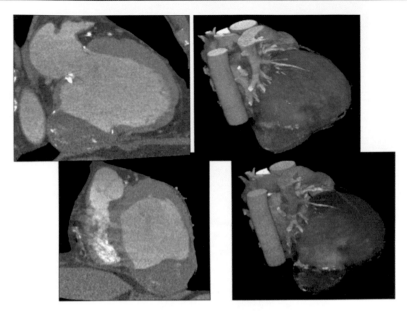

Figure 4.21 Thrombosed left ventricular pseudoaneurysm. This figure shows images of a large, thrombosed saccular pseudoaneurysm of the left ventricle, which measures 7.4 × 7.2 × 4.1. There is global, severe left ventricular dilatation. Involving the inferior and posterior regions of the proximal half of the left ventricle is a saccular-appearing outpouching, which is filled with partially calcified thrombus.

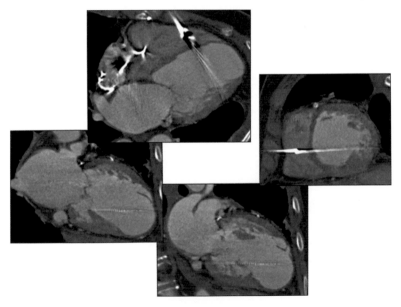

Figure 4.22 Ischemic cardiomyopathy, assessment of scar tissue. This figure shows images of a patient with CAD and ischemic cardiomyopathy and prior coronary bypass surgery, who is evaluated for possible redo open-heart surgery. There are severe calcified atherosclerotic changes of the native coronary arteries and evidence of prior coronary bypass surgery (grafts not shown in the figure). There is moderate left ventricular dilatation and moderate left atrial dilatation. There is thinning of the septal, anteroseptal, and inferoseptal myocardium in the mid and distal segments, consistent with myocardial scar. There is thinning and bulging of the left ventricular apex, consistent with an aneurysm. There is no evidence of thrombus, Pacemaker wires extend into the right atrium and right ventricle.

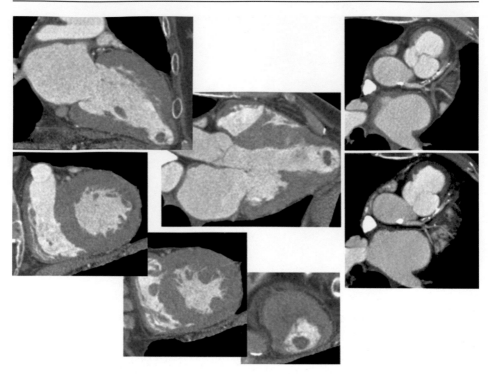

Figure 4.23 Small apical left ventricular aneurysm with thrombus. This figure shows images of a small left ventricular apical aneurysm containing thrombus. Significant accumulation of mixed (calcified and non-calcified) plaque and luminal narrowing is seen in the mid-LAD coronary artery (right panels).

in the diagnosis of myocarditis, guiding of endomyocardial biopsy, and in follow-up.[57] CT imaging is limited (**Figure 4.24**). In contrast to scars related to coronary artery disease, the distribution of the scar tissue does not follow vascular territories and is epicardial rather than endocardial.

4.3.2 Non-Ischemic Atrial and Ventricular Aneurysms and Diverticula

Left ventricular diverticula are congenital outpouchings of the LV cavity with maintained wall structure (**Figures 4.25** and **4.26**). Diverticula can be differentiated from focal aneurysms by the maintained contractility on functional studies, including echocardiography and MRI. Small myocardial crypts are seen in patient with HCM.[58,59] Aneurysmal bulging of the intra-atrial septum and fibrous part of the intraventricular septum can be visualized with CT. However, further assessment of shunt flow requires examination with echocardiography and MRI.

4.3.3 Atrial and Ventricular Thrombus Formation

Atrial and ventricular thrombus formation is associated with various underlying pathologies. Echocardiography is well established in its diagnosis, allowing both identification of the thrombus and underlying wall motion abnormalities. MRI has the advantage of thrombus

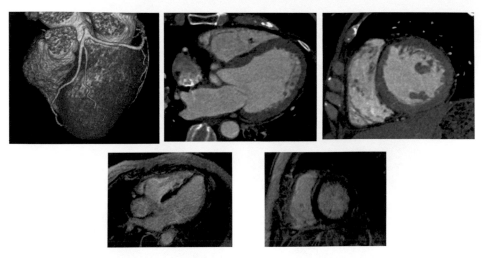

Figure 4.24 Myocarditis. A 42-year-old female presented with symptoms of chest pain and arrhythmia. Clinical features and laboratory tests were consistent with myocarditis. The volume-rendered image (VRI) shows normal coronary arteries. The four-chamber and short-axial images show an area of low density in the epi-myocardium of septal wall. The delayed enhanced CMR images (lower panel) validated the delayed hyperenhancement in the same area.

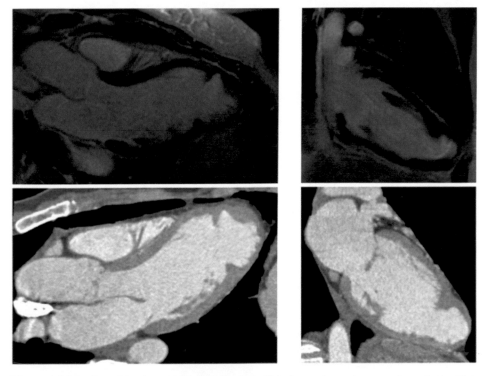

Figure 4.25 Left ventricular apical diverticulum. This figure shows images of a patient with a left ventricular apical diverticulum. MRI and CT images are shown in the upper and lower panels, respectively. At the left ventricular apex, there is a saccular outpouching in communication with the main cavity of the left ventricle. The wall of the outpouching is comprised of myocardial tissue demonstrating systolic contraction on MRI. There is no evidence of fibrosis of calcification of the wall and no thrombus within its cavity.

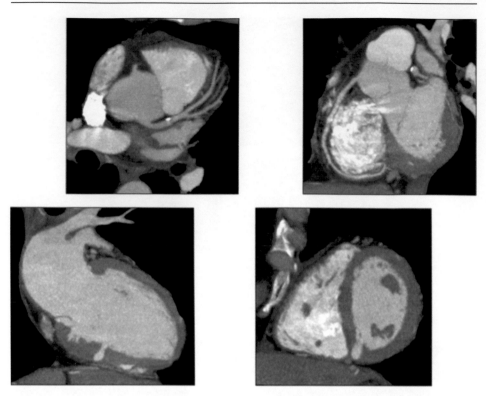

Figure 4.26 Left ventricular diverticulum. This figure shows images of a focal diverticulum of the left ventricular cavity, which extends into the inferior wall near the mid-interventricular septum. There is focal thinning of the left ventricular wall, but the area is surrounded by myocardium. In the differential diagnosis, an incomplete muscular ventricular septal defect (VSD) should be considered. In contrast to post-infarct aneurysms, there is only mild coronary artery of the LAD.

tissue characterization. CT provides good anatomic characterization with the advantage of routine 3-D reconstruction.

Left atrial appendage (LAA) clot is common and frequently associated with atrial fibrillation. With CT it appears as a filling defect in the appendage (**Figure 4.27**).[60] However, slow flow in the LAA as described by transesophageal echocardiography may appear as an LAA filling defect on CT. The appearance depends on the contrast timing, with inhomogeneous, incomplete contrast filling in a hypo-kinetic LAA having similar appearance as thrombus. In these situations, a delayed acquisition can be useful. Right atrial thrombus is less common, seen associated with injury related to the tip of a central venous line and underlying abnormalities of coagulation are often suspected (**Figure 4.28**).

Left ventricular thrombus is often associated with post-infarct aneurysms. Identification is most reliable with MRI and echocardiography, which show thrombus, associated wall motion abnormalities, and in the case of MRI, underlying myocardial scar. CT also reliably demonstrates thrombus (**Figure 4.29**).[61]

4.3.4 Lipomatous Hypertrophy

Lipomatous hypertrophy describes prominent fatty infiltration of the intra-atrial septum (**Figure 4.30**).[62,63]

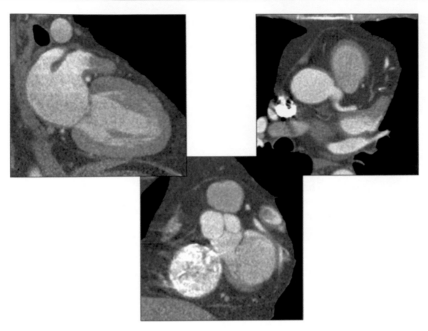

Figure 4.27 Left atrial appendage clot. This figure shows images of a filling defect in the left atrial appendage (LAA), most consistent with clot.

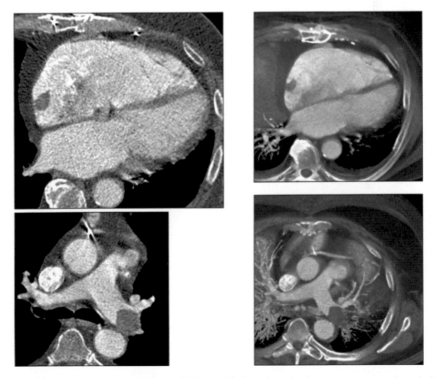

Figure 4.28 Right atrial thrombus. Right atrial thrombus is less common and underlying abnormalities of coagulation are often suspected. In this figure, images of a patient with pulmonary embolism and right atrial thrombus are shown.

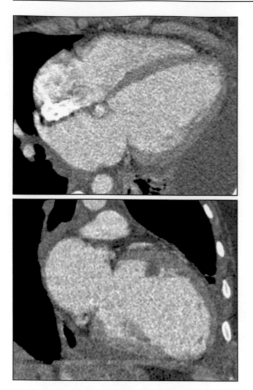

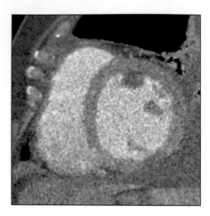

Figure 4.29 Left ventricular thrombus. Although left ventricular thrombus is often associated with post-infarct aneurysms, occasional left ventricular clot without underlying LV dysfunction is found.

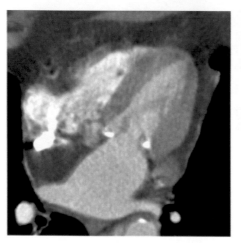

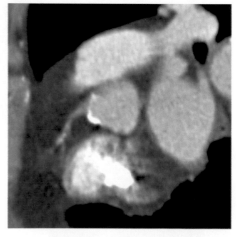

Figure 4.30 Lipomatous hypertrophy of the left atrial septum. Lipomatous hypertrophy describes prominent fatty infiltration of the intra-atrial septum. There is evidence of a mitral valvular annuloplasty ring.

5

Pericardial Disease

The normal pericardium is a thin, double-layered sac surrounding the heart and proximal central vessels (**Figure 5.1**). Together, the visceral/epicardial layer, the parietal layer, and the trivial physiologic amount of fluid, have a normal thickness of about 1–2 mm. The two layers are lined by thin rims of visceral epi-/peri-cardial fat. Identification with imaging modalities is facilitated by these physiologic layers of epicardial and pericardial fat, which provide natural contrast. Echocardiography, MRI, and CT are all well established for the diagnosis of pericardial anatomy.

In the assessment of pericardial disease, functional assessment of cardiac function and flow patterns across the mitral and tricuspid valve relative to the respiratory cycle are critical components. Therefore, echocardiography and MRI are the preferred diagnostic modalities. CT is used in situations, where more detailed anatomic assessment is indicated, e.g. extent and pattern of calcification prior to pericardectomy. Retrospective gating with reconstruction in multiple phases allows limited functional assessment with CT, but the temporal resolution is inferior to echo and MRI. Imaging results need to be evaluated in the context of clinical findings and inflammatory serum markers.[64]

CT allows reliable identification of pericardial anatomy on non–contrast-enhanced scans. CT scans performed with intravenous contrast administration provide additional anatomic information, including associated myocardial disease and evidence of inflammation with pericardial enhancement.

- Congenital or postsurgical absence of the pericardium is identified by complete or focal discontinuity of the pericardial layer (**Figures 5.2** and **5.3**).
- Pericardial thickening can be identified (**Figure 5.4**), and local pattern of thickening and calcification is clearly seen on scans with and without contrast (**Figure 5.5**).
- The identification of pericardial effusion, description of distribution adjacent to the left and right ventricles, quantification of the amount, and basic characteristics of pericardial fluid are possible (**Figures 5.6–5.9**). Indirect evidence of tamponade can be identified.
- Pericardial cysts can be identified defined in relation to adjacent structures (**Figures 5.10** and **5.11**).
- Pericardial primary or metastatic pericardial tumours (Chapter 11) can be described.

Combinations of these anatomic findings are found in specific pericardial disease entities:

- The detection of increased pericardial thickness, especially with pericardial calcium, in combination with conical/tubular deformation of the ventricles, atrial enlargement, and enlargement of the IVC provides evidence of pericardial constriction (**Figures 5.12** and **5.13**). However, these findings do not prove the

DOI: 10.1201/9781003153641-7

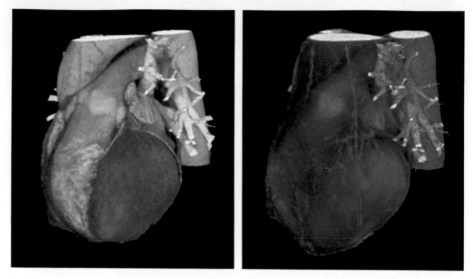

Figure 5.1 Normal pericardium. The normal pericardium, which has a thickness of 1–2 mm, can be delineated over the left and right ventricle. By changing opacity in these volume-rendered images, the heart is seen with (right panel) and without (left panel) the normal pericardium. The thin pericardial sac wraps the ventricles, and the proximal ascending aorta.

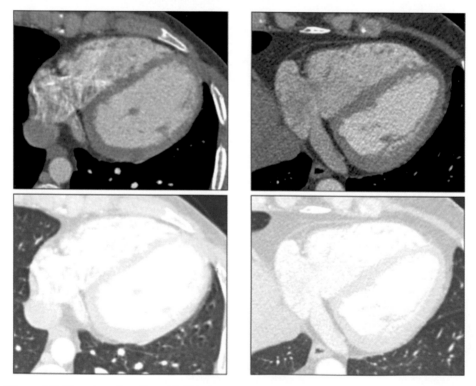

Figure 5.2 Absent pericardium (a). This figure compares normal pericardial anatomy (right panels) with congenital absence of the pericardium (left panels). The relation of the lungs, the pericardial fat, and the pericardium are shown. The image settings in the upper panels are optimized for soft tissue, the lower panels for lung tissue ('lung windows').

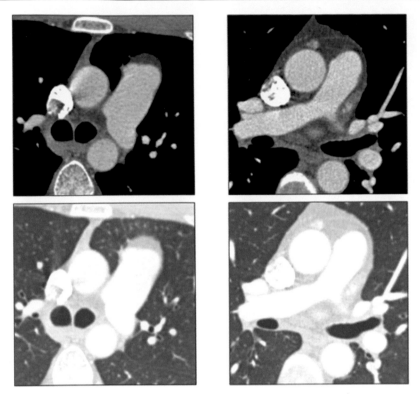

Figure 5.3 Absent pericardium (b). Because the normal pericardium extends to the proximal ascending aorta, the recess between the aorta and pulmonary artery provides further clues to the absence of the pericardium. As shown in this figure, this recess is filled by lung tissue in the patient with absence of the pericardium.

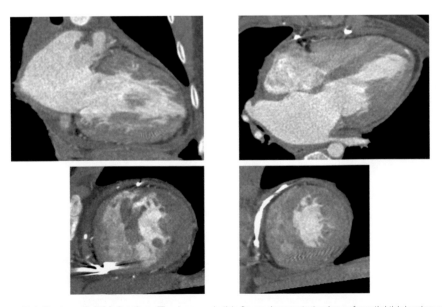

Figure 5.4 Pericardial thickening. The images in this figure demonstrate circumferential thickening and scattered calcification of the pericardium. An epicardial pacer wire is seen adjacent to the right ventricle.

61

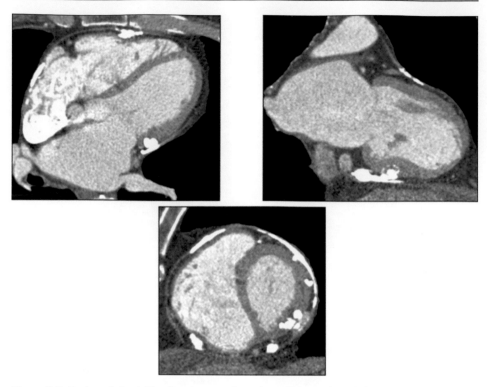

Figure 5.5 Pericardial calcification. Images of a patient with extensive calcification of the pericardium are shown in this image. Calcification of the posterolateral wall appears to extend into the myocardium.

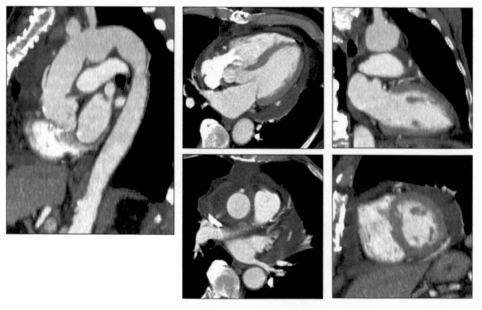

Figure 5.6 Postoperative pericardial effusion (1). This figure shows images of a patient after replacement of the ascending aorta with a supra-coronary graft (left panel). There is a small- to moderate-sized circumferential pericardial effusion without morphologic evidence of tamponade.

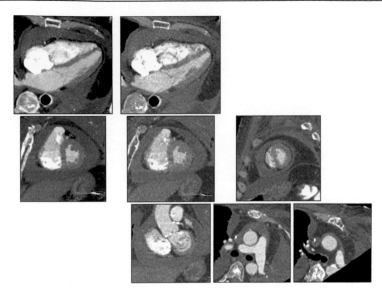

Figure 5.7 Pericardial effusion. The images are obtained from a patient, who presented with shortness of breath 1 month after initiation of Coumadin therapy. The images show normal pericardial thickness with a moderate pericardial effusion. The Hounsfield unit is higher than expected for simple fluid and suggests a haemorrhagic effusion. There is straightening of the interventricular septum and tubular deformity of the left ventricle, suggesting a component of pericardial constriction. The right ventricle is mildly dilated, without evidence of tamponade. Subsequently, surgical pericardectomy was performed. During surgery, a partially organized 1-inch thick layer of circumferential thrombus was removed.

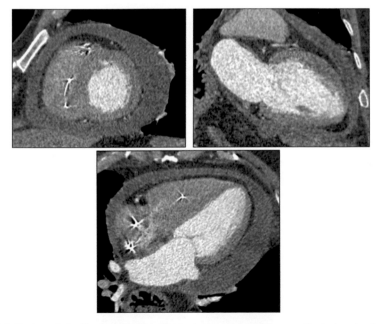

Figure 5.8 Pericardial effusion (2). This figure shows images from a patient who developed fever and cough several days after a pulmonary vein ablation procedure for atrial fibrillation. The CT was performed to evaluate pulmonary vein anatomy. The images show a moderate pericardial effusion with fluid characteristics, which was thought to be an inflammatory response after the ablation (similar to the postcardiotomy or Dressler syndrome).

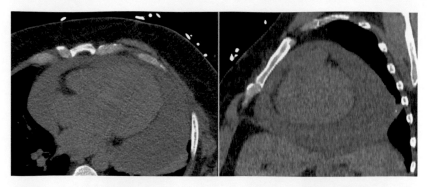

Figure 5.9 Pericardial effusion (3). This figure shows images from a non-contrast CT with a large pericardial effusion, with simple fluid characteristics.

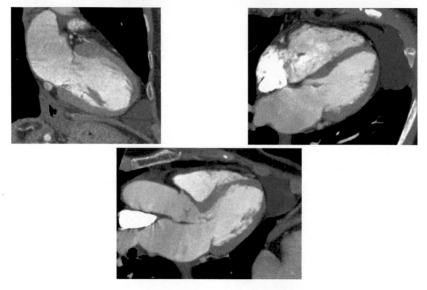

Figure 5.10 Pericardial cyst (1). In this figure, a pericardial cyst over the left ventricular apex is shown. Contrast-enhanced scans help in the differentiation between cyst and normal ventricular cavity.

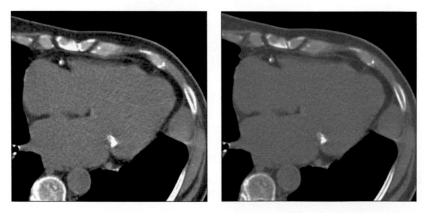

Figure 5.11 Pericardial cyst (2). In these non–contrast-enhanced CTs, a small apical pericardial cyst is identified.

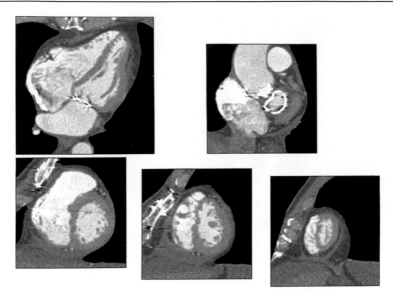

Figure 5.12 Pericardial constriction. This figure shows images of a patient with remote history of mitral valve repair with a prosthetic ring (right upper panel). There is diffuse circumferential thickening of the pericardium measuring up to 5 mm. There is a small amount of pericardial effusion, localized predominantly over the inferior aspect of the right ventricle (lower middle panel). There is tubular deformation of the normal size left and right ventricle (upper left panel). These findings are consistent with pericardial constriction. Confirmation with functional imaging studies e.g. echocardiography or magnetic resonance imaging is required.

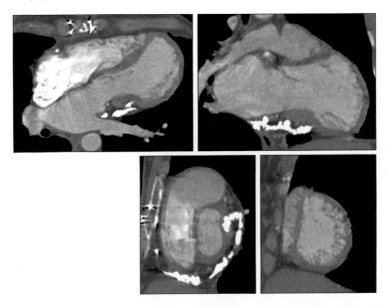

Figure 5.13 Pericardial constriction, prior pericardectomy. Images of a patient with previous history of pericardectomy of the pericardium in the mid to apical segments of the left and right ventricle. There is dense calcification of the thickened, residual pericardium in the basal segments over the inferior wall of the right ventricle, inferior and lateral wall of the left ventricle. The calcification appears to extend into the myocardium in the lateral wall of the left ventricle. There is associated focal tubular deformity of the basal segments of the left ventricle. On 4-D reconstructions, these areas demonstrate the evidence of constriction with normal motion of the mid to distal myocardial segments.

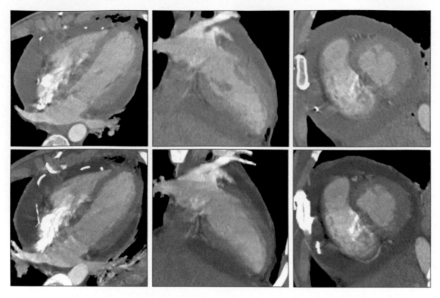

Figure 5.14 Pericardial tamponade. This figure shows images of a patient with recent open-heart surgery for replacement of the aortic root. There is a large pericardial effusion with partial compression of the right atrium. In addition, dilatation of the inferior vena cava was seen. These findings are consistent with tamponade.

presence of constrictive physiology, and on the other hand constrictive physiology can be found in the absence of obvious anatomic abnormalities.

- Findings consistent with tamponade are right ventricular collapse or indirect signs including enlargement of the hepatic veins (**Figures 5.14** and **5.15**). However, functional assessment is critical and is the strength of echocardiography and MRI.

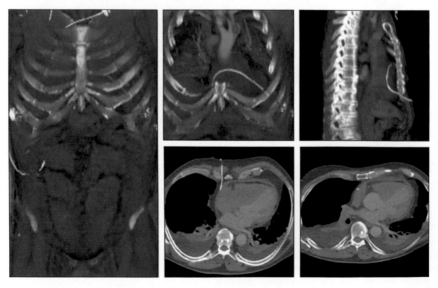

Figure 5.15 Pericardial tamponade. This figure shows images of a patient after pericardiocentesis for a large pericardial effusion with tamponade. The position of the drainage catheter is shown. The right lower panel shows the tip of the drain in the residual effusion. Additional small, bilateral pleural effusions are seen.

- Pericardial enhancement after contrast injection is consistent with pericarditis (**Figure 5.16**). Identification of pericardial enhancement with dedicated T2 ('edema'-weighted) and delayed contrast-enhanced ('scar') MRI imaging is a recent area of interest. In patients with recurrent pericarditis, it may allow the understanding of temporal patterns of disease activity and impact of pharmacological intervention. [65–67]

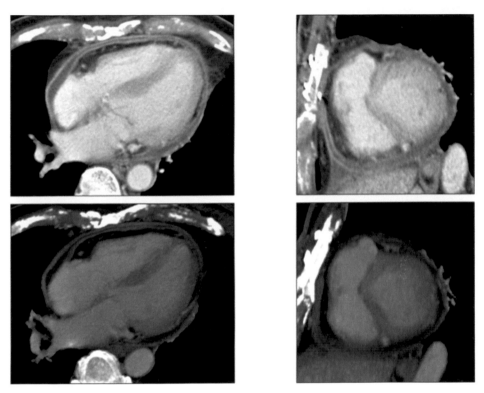

Figure 5.16 Pericardial enhancement. CT scans after contrast administration can provide information about the possible inflammatory nature of a pericardial process. Contrast enhancement of the pericardial layers, as shown in this figure, is consistent with pericarditis.

6

Valvular Heart Disease

The assessment of valvular heart disease is a strength of echocardiography and magnetic resonance imaging, because of their ability to assess anatomic and functional detail. Imaging with CT is limited secondary to the lower temporal resolution. However, advances in scanner technology have improved the assessment of valvular structures, and dynamic '4-D' reconstruction of retrospective gated CT acquisition with fast multidetector scanners can provide insight into valvular function.[68]

Imaging of the aortic valve allows differentiation between normal tricuspid (**Figure 2.10**), bicuspid (**Figures 6.1** and **6.2**), and quatrocuspid (**Figure 6.3**) aortic valve anatomy. CT can precisely describe the extent and location of valvular calcification, which correlates with severity of aortic stenosis (**Figure 6.4**). CT allows identification of sub-aortic membranes (**Figure 6.5**). CT can also identify anatomic correlates of aortic insufficiency (**Figure 6.6**).

Thickening and calcification of the mitral valve leaflets, which are often associated with mitral stenosis (**Figure 6.7**), and calcification at the mitral valve annulus (**Figure 6.8**) can be described. In patients with mitral valve prolapse, the typical systolic displacement of the mitral valve leaflets can be demonstrated (**Figure 6.9**). CT has recently been described in the assessment of mitral annular disjunction.[69]

Assessment of the pulmonary valve is possible and has recently been described in the context of transcatheter pulmonary valve replacement (**Figure 6.10**).

In patients with Ebstein's anomaly, the displacement of the tricuspid valve towards the right ventricle can be described (**Figure 6.11**).

Reliable assessment of vegetations remains a strength of echocardiography. 4-D CT can identify vegetations (**Figures 6.12** and **6.13**).[70,71]

A strength of CT is postoperative evaluation after valve repair or replacement. Correct positioning of the prosthetic ring or prosthetic valve can be assessed (**Figures 6.14–6.17**), and complications including valve dehiscence can be identified (**Figure 6.18**).[168,169]

CT plays an important role for planning of transcatheter interventional procedures including TAVR (see Chapter 7).

DOI: 10.1201/9781003153641-8

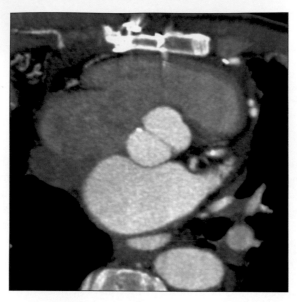

Figure 6.1 Bicuspid aortic valve. This figure shows an example of a bicuspid aortic valve. There is fusion of the left and right coronary cusp. The identification of the non-coronary cusp is guided by its location between the left and right atrium in the short-axis view and of course the lack of coronary ostia.

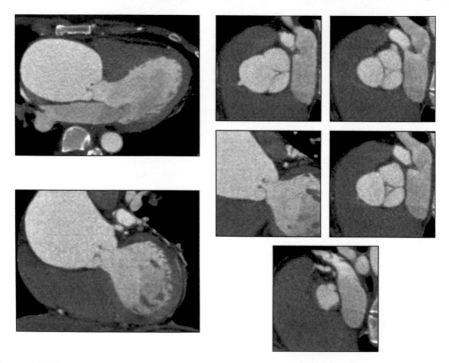

Figure 6.2 Bicuspid aortic valve with partial fusion of the non- and left coronary cusp. This figure shows images of a bicuspid aortic valve with partial fusion of the non-coronary and left coronary cusp. There is eccentric prominence of the right-coronary cusp and massive dilatation of the ascending aorta with severe effacement of the sinotubular junction. The lack of coaptation of the leaflets in diastole (middle panels) is consistent with aortic insufficiency. Both bicuspid valve anatomy and aortic insufficiency were confirmed by echocardiography.

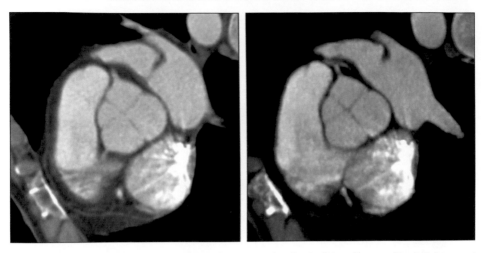

Figure 6.3 **Quatrocuspid aortic valve.** This aortic valve has four leaflets, with a small leaflet interposed between the left and right coronary cusps.

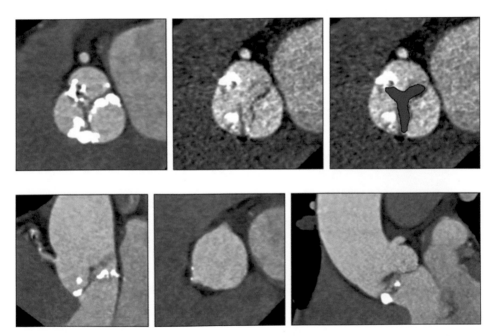

Figure 6.4 **Severe aortic stenosis with aortic valve calcification.** This figure shows images of a patient with a history of severe aortic stenosis, who underwent prior valvuloplasty. There is severe calcification of the aortic valve leaflets, in particular at the raphe between the left and right coronary cusp (10 o'clock position). There was moderate residual aortic stenosis by echocardiography. Planimetry was attempted in the systolic CT image (middle upper panel) and resulted in a valve area of 1.6 cm². However, measurements are often limited by calcium volume-averaging ('blooming') artefact. The lower panels show the origin of the coronary arteries from the corresponding sinuses (RCA ostium: left lower panel; LM ostium: right lower panel). The middle lower panel shows a cross-section of the aorta at the level of the coronary artery origin (RCA ostium: 7 o'clock; LM ostium 12 o'clock).

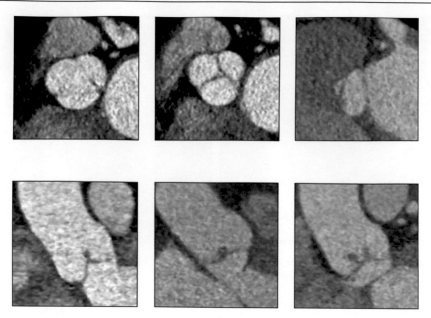

Figure 6.5 Sub-aortic membrane. The differential diagnosis of aortic stenosis is flow obstruction in the left ventricular outflow tract caused by a sub-aortic membrane. These figures show a membrane of the anterior aspect of the outflow tract, below the valve level in the area of the non-coronary cusp (lower middle and right panels).

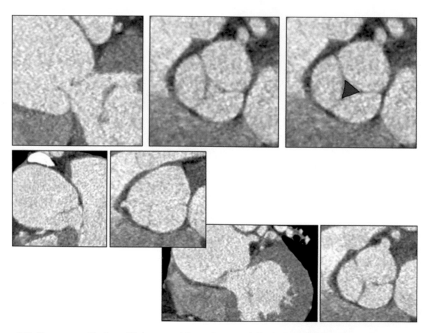

Figure 6.6 Severe aortic insufficiency with prolapse of the left coronary cusp. This figure shows images of a patient with severe aortic insufficiency. There is mild, asymmetric prominence of the left coronary cusp (upper middle panel, origin of the left main coronary artery at 1 o'clock). This is associated with prolapse of the left coronary cups (left upper panel). There is incomplete coaptation of the aortic valve leaflets in diastole (residual opening shown in red in the right upper panel). There is no calcification of the aortic valve leaflets. The aortic root is dilated with severe effacement of the sinotubular junction.

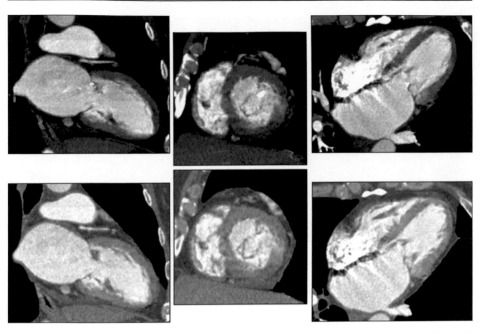

Figure 6.7 Mitral valve calcification in mitral stenosis. This figure shows images of a patient with chronic atrial fibrillation and mitral stenosis. The left atrium shows moderate-to-severe dilatation without evidence of clot. There is thickening and calcification of the mitral valve leaflets compatible with mitral stenosis.

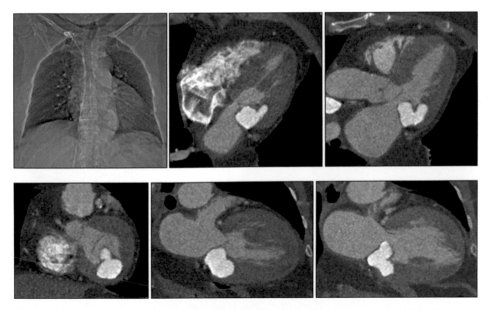

Figure 6.8 Severe mitral annular calcification. This figure shows images of a high-attenuation lesion, arising within the posterior mitral annulus and extends into the posterior left ventricular wall. The findings are most consistent with mitral annular calcification.

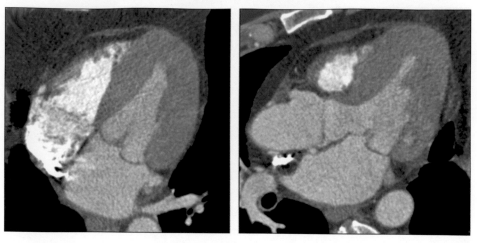

Figure 6.9 Mitral valve prolapse. The images show mild thickening of the mitral valve leaflets. There is prolapse of both leaflets during systole with bulging towards the left atrium. There is concentric left ventricular hypertrophy involving the left ventricle.

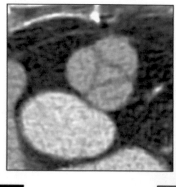

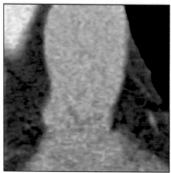

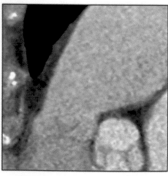

Figure 6.10 Pulmonary valve, status post-valvuloplasty. This figure shows images of a patient with a history of pulmonary valve stenosis and prior valvuloplasty. The thickened valve leaflets are well seen in the upper panel. The lower panels illustrate dilatation of the central pulmonary artery.

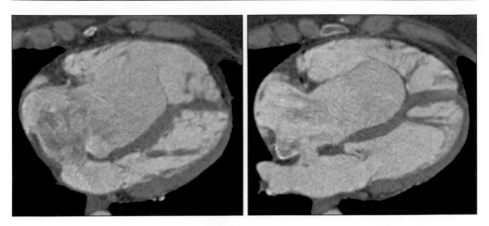

Figure 6.11 Ebstein's anomaly. Ebstein's anomaly describes the apical displacement of the tricuspid valve insertion towards the right ventricle. The images show severe dilatation of the right ventricle and right atrium. Displacement of the septal component of the tricuspid valve from the normal position at the atrioventricular septum towards the right ventricle, consistent with changes of Ebstein's anomaly.

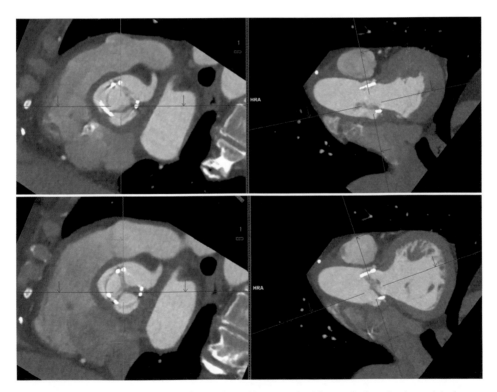

Figure 6.12 Endocarditis (1). This figure shows images of a bio-prosthetic valve in systole (upper panels) and diastole (lower panels). There is a linear density extending during systole into the aortic root, consistent with a vegetation.

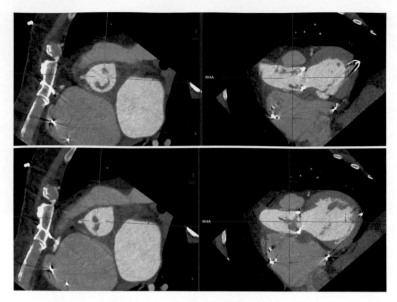

Figure 6.13 Endocarditis (2). This figure shows images of another bio-prosthetic valve. Again, images are in systole (upper panels) and diastole (lower panels). There is a nodular density extending during systole into the aortic root, consistent with a vegetation.

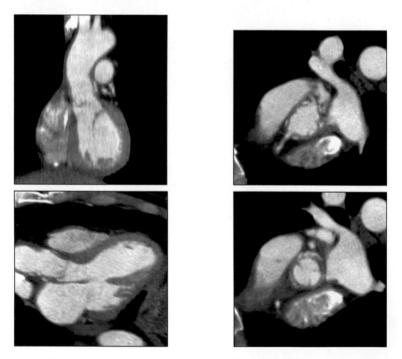

Figure 6.14 Aortic root replacement with a composite graft including re-suspension of the native aortic valve (David procedure). This figure shows evidence of aortic root replacement with a composite graft including re-suspension of the native aortic valve into a surgical tube graft of the proximal ascending aorta (David procedure). The right panels show the re-implanted coronary arteries (upper panel, 1 and 8 o'clock positions) and the re-suspended valve (lower panel).

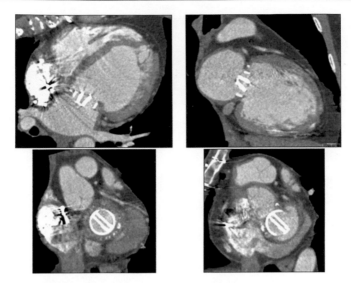

Figure 6.15 Mitral valve replacement with mechanical valve. This figure shows images of a patient after mitral valve replacement. The cardiac chambers show mild dilatation of the left ventricle. There is replacement of the mitral valve with a mechanical prosthesis. The tilting discs are well seen.

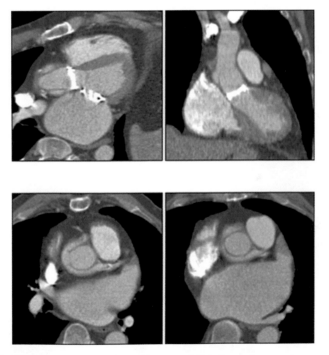

Figure 6.16 Mitral valve and aortic valve replacement. This figure shows an images of a patient after mitral and aortic valve replacement and coronary bypass surgery. There is left atrial dilatation and a filling defect in the left atrial appendage consistent with thrombus or slow flow. There is evidence of mitral valve replacement with a mechanical valve. There is evidence of a valved conduit graft of the ascending thoracic aorta, with a mechanical aortic valve. The coronary arteries are re-implanted in the lateral segment of the grafted ascending aorta with an interposed graft dividing into two limbs, connecting to the native coronary arteries. Beyond the graft of the ascending aorta, the native aorta has normal dimensions.

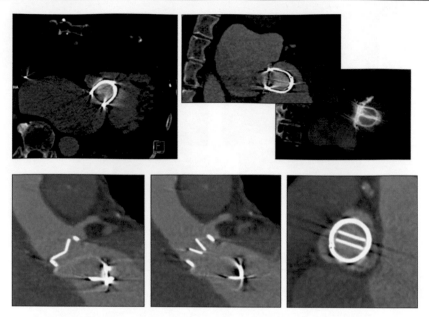

Figure 6.17 Mitral valve (ball-in-cage) and aortic valve (tilting-disc) replacement. This figure shows images of a patient after mitral and aortic valve replacement. The upper panels show a ball-in-cage valve (Starr-Edwards) in the mitral position. The metal struts of the cage are well seen. However, the ball is not well visualized. The lower panels show diastolic (left lower panel) and systolic (middle and right lower panels) of the aortic valve prosthesis. The position of the tilting discs is well seen.

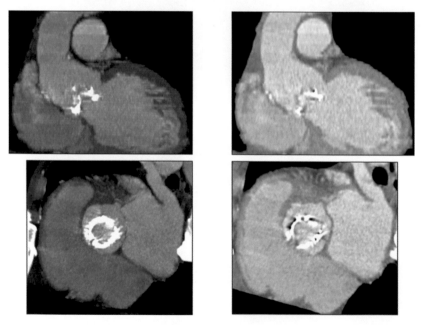

Figure 6.18 Aortic valve dehiscence. This figure shows images of a patient with remote aortic valve replacement and suspected endocarditis. There is a bioprosthetic Carpentier Edwards aortic valve and supracoronary graft of the ascending aorta. There is increased size of the aortic root (5.2 cm) with separation of the valve ring at the left and right sinuses of Valsalva. During surgery, an aortic periprosthetic leak was identified and replacement with a homograft performed.

7

CT Planning and Guidance for Transcatheter Interventions

Although the role of CT in the diagnosis of valvular disease is limited secondary to the limited functional and physiological (flow) data, CT has a prominent role for the detailed anatomical assessment of eligibility and for planning of transcatheter structural and valvular heart procedures, exemplified in the experience of TAVR (**Figures 7.1** and **7.2**).[72]

CT allows unlimited reconstructions of oblique planes through structures with a complex 3-D anatomy or orientation. Therefore, these structures can be viewed from any angle after image acquisition, whereas review of standard 2-D-tomographic techniques such as TTE or TEE is limited to the echocardiographic windows acquired. Analysis can be performed on standard CT workstations with conventional software, but dedicated software are increasingly available and simplify the analyses and may shorten the learning curve.[73]

TAVR planning includes evaluation of the anatomic suitability of aortic annulus size and vascular access anatomy, which facilitates the selection of the correct prosthesis size. MDCT is considered the most reliable modality for identification of anatomic features that are contraindications for TAVR and/or associated with increased risk of complications. MDCT acquisition protocols for planning TAVR should include a cardiac scan including the ascending aorta and a vascular overview of the entire thoracoabdominal aorta including the subclavian vessels and the femoral artery bifurcation. In general ECG-gated spiral scanning with wide pulsing and retrospectively gated reconstruction is recommended for the heart and aortic root/annulus. Measurements at the annulus and root are typically performed in systolic reconstructions (**Figures 7.3** and **7.4**). The vascular overview is typically acquired with non-gated protocols. Alternatively, a single high-pitch spiral acquisition protocol has been reported to provide good results with reduced contrast and radiation exposure.[74]

In contrast to surgical aortic valve replacement, where the prosthesis size is selected under direct vision, TAVR relies on imaging for sizing. Assessments of aortic annulus measurements are performed on double oblique transverse views of the aortic annulus. The annulus defines as a virtual plane through the three inferior insertion points of the aortic valve leaflets, and is typically oval-shaped (**Figures 7.4** and **7.5**).

The non-circular dimensions and in particular the long-axis diameter cannot be fully appreciated or quantified on 2-D TTE/TEE. Consequently, sizing by TTE/TEE leads more frequently to undersizing, which causes aortic regurgitation when compared to sizing by MDCT.[75-77] The degree of calcification of the aortic leaflets and the anterior mitral valve leaflet at the level of the aortic annulus area is quantified using the Agatston score, optimally on non-contrast scans (**Figure 7.5**). Dense aortic root calcification is a major determinant of paravalvular leakage. In contrast, low levels of aortic valve calcification may contribute to device dislodgement during TAVR.

Accuracy of transcatheter aortic valve replacement (TAVI) is increased when the catheter laboratory C-arm is in the correct position separating the three aortic sinuses

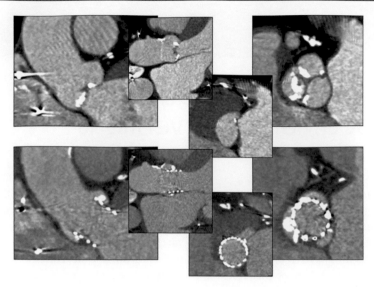

Figure 7.1 **Transcatheter aortic valve replacement, stent valve (a).** These images and those in the following figure show a patient that underwent aortic valve replacement. This figure compares pre- and post-operative images of the aortic valve and aortic root (upper panels = pre-; lower panels = post-procedure). There is dense calcification of the aortic valve leaflets, consistent with the patient's history of severe aortic stenosis. The lower panels show the stent/valve well seated in the aortic root, displacing the calcified leaflets against the aortic wall.

and showing them all in the same plane. The optimal projection of the C-arm can be determined from pre-procedural CT instead of having to perform multiple catheter injections in a trial-and-error approach (**Figure 7.6**).[78]

For evaluation of vascular access, the minimum vessel diameter and also the degree and distribution of calcification and tortuosity are considered. The transfemoral route is preferred but in cases where it is not accessible all potential alternative routes may be evaluated on the same scan including trans-subclavian, trans-apical, and direct aortic access (**Figures 7.7** and **7.8**).

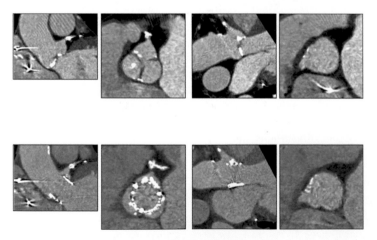

Figure 7.2 **Transapical aortic valve replacement, stent valve (b).** This figure compares pre- and post-operative images of the coronary ostia (upper panels = pre-; lower panels = post-procedure). The relationship of the stent/valve to the left main ostium (left two panels) and right coronary ostium (right two panels) is demonstrated.

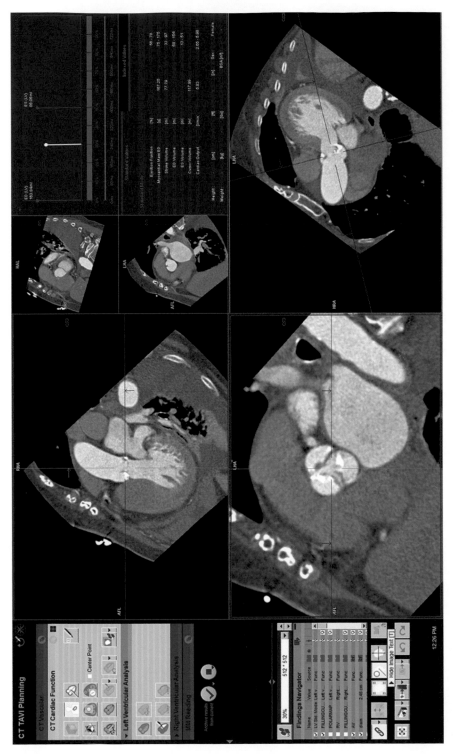

Figure 7.3 **Aortic valve stenosis with star-shaped opening of leaflet tips (systolic reconstruction).** This figure shows images of a patient with severe aortic stenosis. Image plane at the leaflet tips shows the severely restricted star-shaped opening.

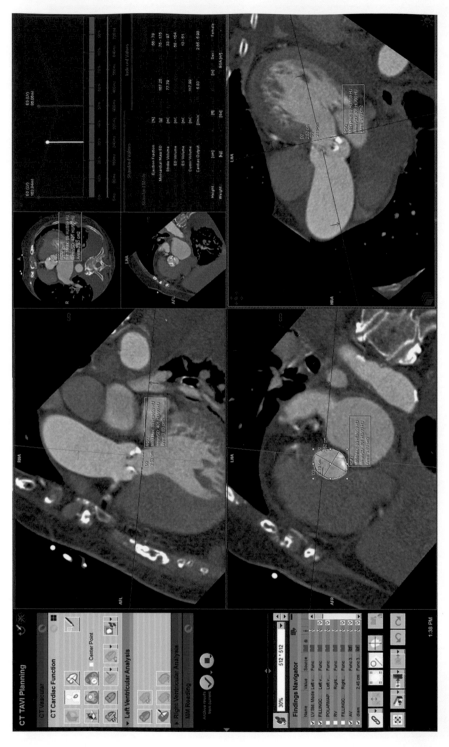

Figure 7.4 Analysis of annular dimensions. This figure shows images reconstructed manually at the lowest level of insertion of the aortic valve leaflets. Diameter and area measurements are shown in the left lower panel.

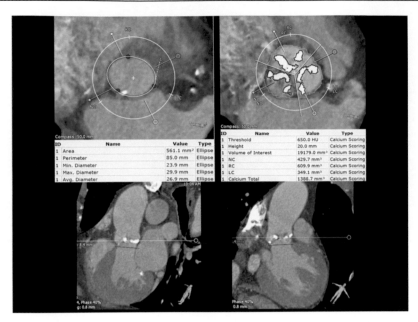

Figure 7.5 Semi-automated analysis and valve calcium scoring. Rapid measurement of all dimensions of the aortic annulus for sizing and of calcification of the leaflets can be performed with dedicated software.

After TAVR, CT allows evaluation of stent frame distention and apposition to native tissue and may reveal the unanticipated causes of poor patient recovery. Post-procedural CT also allows to evaluate hypo-attenuated leaflet thickening (HALT) and associated decreased leaflet motion hypo-attenuation affecting motion (HAM) (**Figure 7.9**).[79]

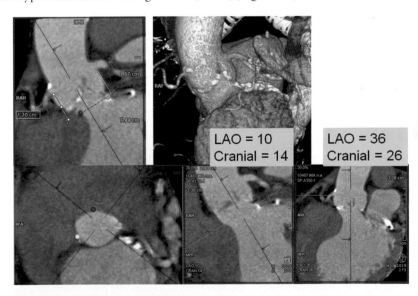

Figure 7.6 Coronary height and rotation. A low origin of the coronary ostia above the aortic annulus is associated with a risk of coronary obstruction when the calcified aortic leaflets are displaced by the TAVR prosthesis. The optimal C-arm angulation to facilitate positioning of the TAVR prosthesis can be determined prior to the procedure on MDCT.

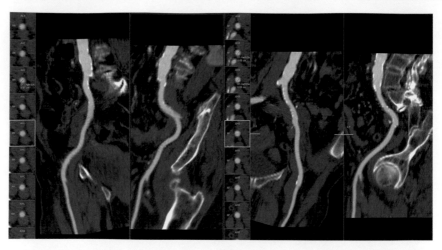

Figure 7.7 Iliac centreline. Dedicated software allows rapid semi-automated centreline extraction of the right and left iliac and femoral arteries with one-click display of the 3-D anatomy, diameter, tortuosity, and calcium distribution and interrogation of short-axis images at any point of interest.

The advantages of planning TAVR procedures with MDCT apply also to other percutaneous procedures including left atrial appendage closure and the developing field of percutaneous mitral and tricuspid valve replacement.[80,81] MDCT allows a detailed evaluation of the dynamic shape and dimensions of the mitral valve annulus throughout the cardiac cycle and various access routes may be assessed (**Figure 7.10**). Similarly, the anatomic features that may impact on the choice whether or not to perform a left atrial appendage closure and on selection of the optimal device are also clearly seen on MDCT (**Figure 7.11**).

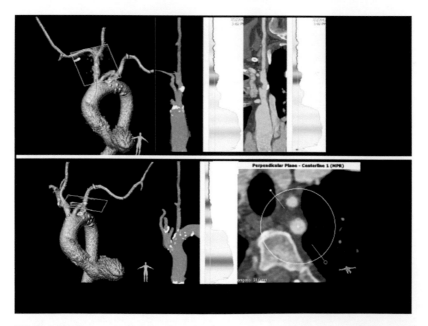

Figure 7.8 Subclavian centreline. Dedicated software allows rapid centreline extraction display and interrogation on 3-D, longitudinal and short-axis images of the trans-subclavian arterial access routes.

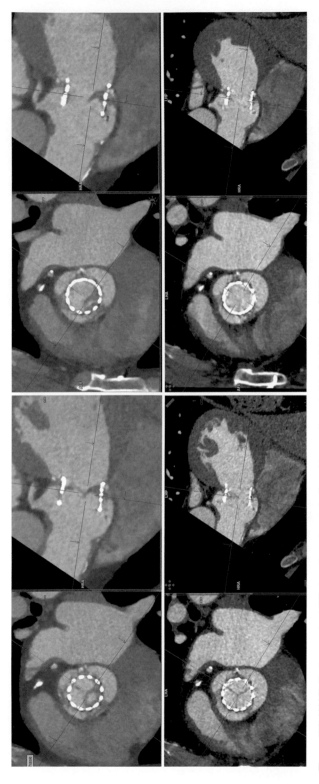

Figure 7.9 HALT. Post-procedural CT also allows for evaluation of hypo-attenuated leaflet thickening (HALT) and associated decreased leaflet motion hypo-attenuation affecting motion (HAM). The upper panels show thickening of the right-facing leaflet 2 months after TAVR. Leaflet thickening disappears after anticoagulation as seen in the lower panels.

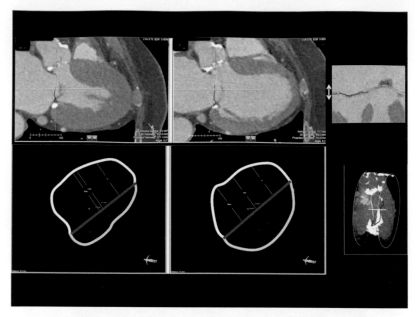

Figure 7.10 Mitral valve. CT is useful for procedure planning of transcatheter mitral valve replacement. Dedicated software allows a detailed evaluation of the mitral annulus throughout the cardiac cycle. The shapes of the annulus and the mitral valve leaflets are shown during systole (left) and diastole (right).

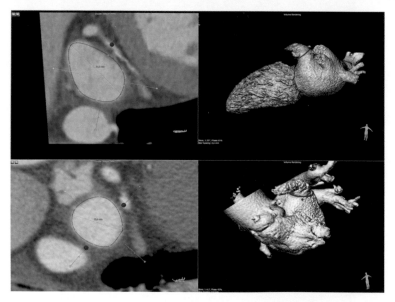

Figure 7.11 Left atrial appendage (LAA). 3-D imaging techniques such as CT are very useful for evaluating the anatomical factors relevant to planning novel procedures, such as left atrial appendage (LAA) occlusion. In these two examples, the shape of the LAA can be seen on the volume-rendered images (right) where the inflow of the LAA is indicated by a red circle. The 2-D images on the left are short-axis view planes showing the shape of the inflow of the LAA and corresponding measurements of area and maximum diameter. In the first case (top row), the 'windsock' shape of the LAA shows a dominant tail of sufficient length relative to the ostium size to allow LAA occlusion. The acute angle change from the inflow to the tail of the appendage in the second case (bottom row), the so-called 'chicken wing' shape is not in ideal anatomy for LAA occlusion.

8

Coronary Arterial and Venous Disease

MDCT imaging with modern CT systems allows comprehensive assessment of coronary anatomy (**Figure 8.1**).[82,83] Non–contrast-enhanced scans (CT calcium scoring) allow an assessment of calcified plaque burden and allow to assess future risk of cardiovascular events in selected asymptomatic patient populations.[84] Indications for contrast-enhanced protocols (CT angiography, CTA) in symptomatic patients include the evaluation of suspected obstructive coronary artery disease (CAD), bypass graft disease, and certain coronary stents. CTA is also applied to the assessment of non-atherosclerotic CAD, such as coronary anomalies, coronary muscle bridge, and coronary aneurysm.[25]

8.1 Coronary Artery Disease

8.1.1 Atherosclerotic Coronary Artery Disease

8.1.1.1 Non-stenotic, subclinical atherosclerosis

Atherosclerotic plaque accumulation in the vessel wall begins long before the development of angiographic stenosis. Most acute coronary events are initiated by rupture or erosion of mildly stenotic but vulnerable (high-risk) lesions.[85] Modern atherosclerosis imaging therefore evaluates overall plaque burden and plaque characteristics as predictors of future cardiovascular risk. Non-enhanced CT imaging (CT calcium scoring) only allows for the assessment of calcified plaque, while contrast-enhanced CTA allows differentiation of calcified and non-calcified plaque.

8.1.1.2 Calcium scoring

The identification of coronary arterial calcification is a sign of chronic atherosclerotic changes. Advanced stenotic lesions causing stable angina pectoris often demonstrate dense calcifications. In contrast, high-risk culprit lesions causing acute coronary events are frequently non-calcified or show microcalcification by histology.[86] CT examinations performed without contrast administration are very sensitive in detecting and quantitating coronary arterial calcification (**Figures 8.2** and **8.3**), but significantly underestimate total atherosclerotic plaque burden (calcified and non-calcified plaque) (**Figures 8.3** and **8.4**). Total calcium load in the coronary tree can be quantified using one of several calcium scoring algorithms, including the traditional Agaston score,[87] volume scoring, and mass scoring. Standardized scan and scoring protocols have been developed for MDCT, with acceptable reproducibility.[88]

DOI: 10.1201/9781003153641-10

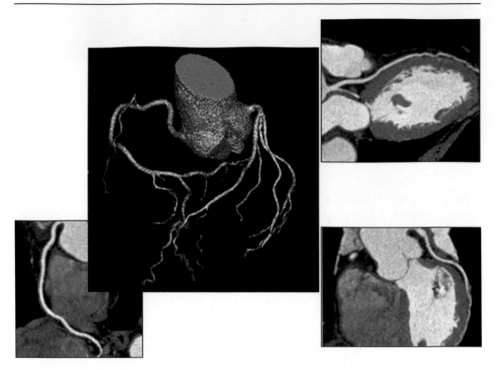

Figure 8.1 Normal coronary anatomy. The VRI image in the centre shows the course of the arteries and side branches. The small images show curved multi-planar reformation (MPR) images of the right coronary artery (RCA, left lower panel), left circumflex coronary artery (LCX, right lower panel), and left anterior descending coronary artery (LAD, right upper panel). There is no evidence of luminal stenosis or atherosclerotic plaque accumulation.

The predictive value of the overall calcium score for future coronary events has been established and is the basis for clinical use.[89,90] Clinical guidelines consider coronary calcium scoring appropriate for selected intermediate risk asymptomatic persons, but clinical use remains limited.[84] Dynamic changes in the calcium volume score during pharmacological therapy have been examined in serial clinical CT trials, but the results are inconsistent.[91,92]

8.1.1.3 Contrast-enhanced CTA for plaque imaging

Similar to intravascular ultrasound (IVUS), contrast-enhanced CT scans allow differentiation of lumen and vessel wall, and identification of both calcified and non-calcified plaque.[93,94] The frequent presence of significant plaque burden in segments without significant luminal stenosis (**Figures 8.5** and **8.6**) is explained by the associated outward expansion of the vessel wall (expansive remodelling), maintaining luminal dimension.[95,96] Non-calcified plaque can be further characterized on the basis of mean Hounsfield unit (HU) number. High-risk plaque features include: low attenuation plaque (less than 30 HU), positive remodelling, spotty calcification, and the 'napkin ring sign.'[97] Occasionally small, contrast-filled cavities of the coronary wall can be identified with CT (**Figure 8.7**). These have an appearance similar

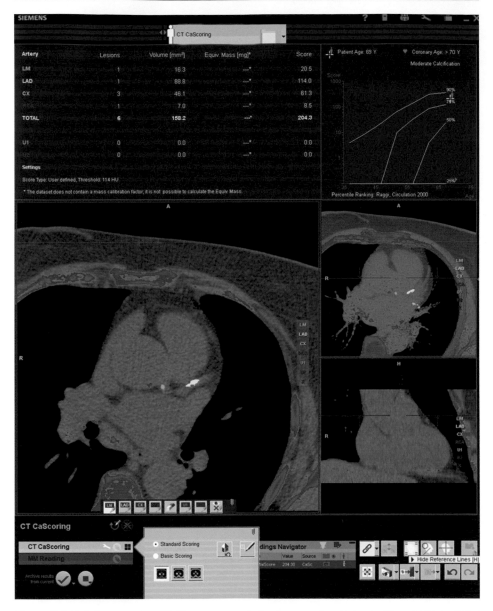

Figure 8.2 Calcium scoring (1). These screenshots show results obtained with a modern clinical scoring software. The non–contrast-enhanced 'calcium scoring' image of a patient with a calcification in the left main (green marker) and proximal left anterior descending coronary artery (yellow marker) (central panel). In the upper part of the images, the results are summarized in a table (left) and relative to a reference population (nomogram).

to penetrating ulcerations in other vessels (e.g. aorta) and are most consistent with previous plaque rupture.

Clinical trials describe the relationship between CT findings and clinical endpoints/ outcome. Low-attenuation plaque and positive vessel remodelling independently predicted subsequent development of acute coronary syndrome.[98,99]

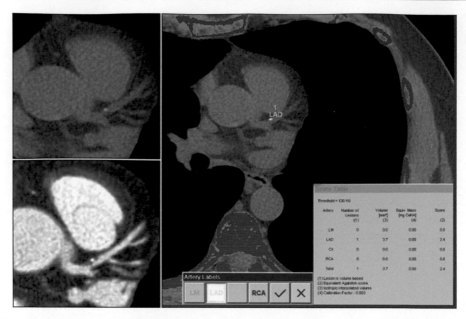

Figure 8.3 Calcium scoring (2). The right panel shows a non–contrast-enhanced 'calcium scoring' image of a patient with a small calcification in the proximal left anterior descending coronary artery (LAD). The calcification is identified by its Hounsfield value above 130 and colour coded. The comparison of the non–contrast-enhanced image (left upper panel) and contrast-enhanced image (left lower panel) shows that the calcified plaque is part of a larger non-calcified plaque.

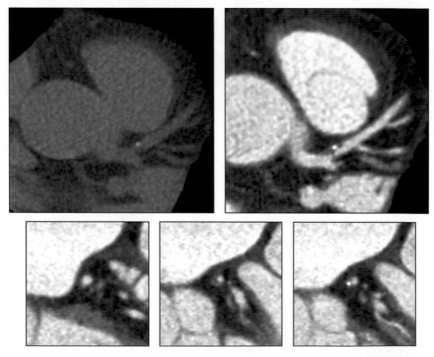

Figure 8.4 Calcified and non-calcified plaque. Comparison of a non–contrast-enhanced image (left upper panel) and contrast-enhanced images (right upper panel and lower panels) demonstrate that the calcified plaque is only part of a larger partially calcified plaque.

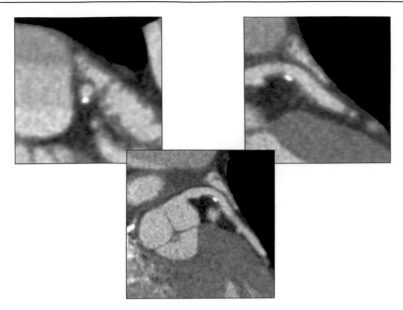

Figure 8.5 Arterial remodelling. Longitudinal and cross-sectional (left upper panel) images showing mild, partially calcified plaque accumulation of the proximal LAD without significant stenosis. Plaque accumulation is not associated with significant stenosis because of expansion of the vessel area (expansive/positive remodelling).

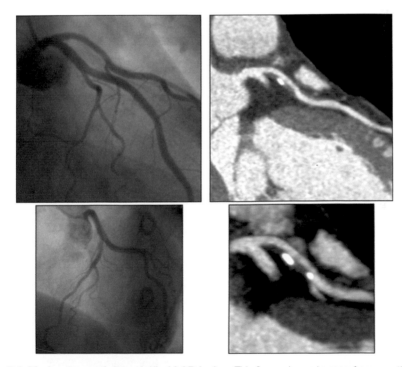

Figure 8.6 Moderate, partially calcified LAD lesion. This figure shows images from a patient with atypical chest pain. Partially calcified plaque in the proximal LAD with mild angiographic stenosis but about 50% cross-sectional narrowing in the diseased segment. The corresponding angiogram confirms mild, non-obstructive luminal stenosis.

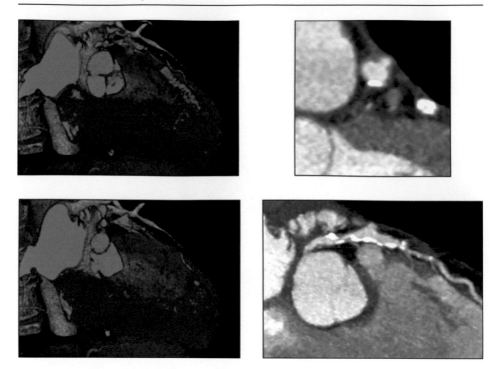

Figure 8.7 Suspected plaque rupture, penetrating ulceration. In this patient, there is mild ectasia of the proximal LAD. In this enlarged segment (right upper panel), there is a non-calcified plaque with a focal cavity of the artery lumen. These small contrast-filled cavities of the coronary wall have an appearance similar to penetrating ulcerations in other vessels (e.g. aorta) and are most consistent with prior plaque rupture, with the now empty necrotic core (lipid pool) areas gaining communication with the artery lumen. Intravascular ultrasound studies have described similar findings, both in the acute and chronic settings.

However, the most rigorous data has accumulated describing the prognostic value of plaque burden.[100–102] Strata of 'absent CAD', 'non-obstructive CAD' (worst stenosis < 50%), or 'obstructive CAD' demonstrated incremental increases in the risk of future major adverse cardiac events (MACE).[103]

8.1.1.4 Stenotic CAD coronary CTA in symptomatic patients

Challenges for coronary CTA are the small size of coronary arteries, coronary calcification, and the fast motion during the cardiac cycle. Large coronary segments with minimal motion, such as the left main (LM) coronary artery and proximal portions of the left anterior descending artery (LAD), are more reliably visualized than segments with more pronounced motion, including parts of the right coronary artery (RCA) and left circumflex coronary artery (LCX), and smaller segments. Coronary arterial motion varies during the cardiac cycle, and individual arteries reach peak velocity at different times during the cardiac cycle. Minimal motion artefact is typically seen in diastolic windows (70–75% RR interval). A second window with limited motion is found in systole (about 30–35% RR interval). Image reconstruction at multiple phases in the cardiac cycle can be very helpful in selected

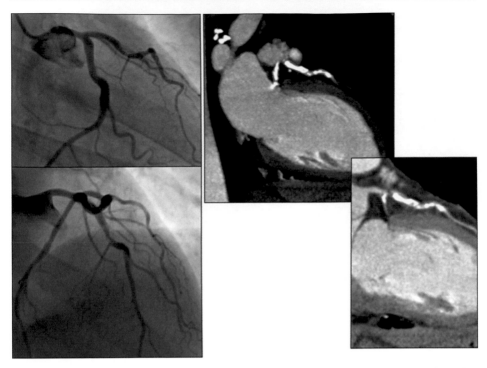

Figure 8.8 Limitation of coronary CTA: Calcium blooming artefact. This figure shows angiographic images from a patient with angiographically moderate luminal stenosis of the proximal LAD (left panels). The CT images (right panels) demonstrate severe calcified atherosclerotic plaque accumulation of the entire proximal LAD. 'Calcium blooming'/volume averaging artefact precludes precise assessment of luminal stenosis/patency with CTA.

patients.[104] Another limitation of CTA is related to coronary arterial calcification, which is a hallmark of advance atherosclerotic disease. The 'blooming' (or "volume average") effect of coronary calcification can result in potential false-positive detection or overestimation of luminal stenosis, and can cause difficulties in assessing adjacent non-calcified plaque structures (**Figure 8.8**). Advances in scanner technology have reduced but not eliminated this artefact.

Clinical trials and experience have demonstrated very high negative predictive values of CT, which allow reliable exclusion of CAD in low- or intermediate-risk patients (**Figure 8.9**). In contrast, the positive predictive value for the detection of significant luminal stenosis is more limited. CTA allows to differentiate mild and severe stenosis (**Figures 8.10–8.19**). Because of the limited spatial resolution and relatively wide confidence interval, it is recommended to report severity of stenosis in broad categories (0%, 1–24%, 25–49%, 50–69%, 70–99%, 100%).[97,105] Meta-analyses of multi-centre CTA trials demonstrate a high diagnostic accuracy to identify patients with ≥50% stenoses by quantitative coronary analysis (QCA), with a pooled area under the curve (AUC) of 0.99.[106,107] However, assessment of stenosis severity in individual coronary arterial lesions is more limited. In the study by Meijboom et al.,[108] sensitivity for detecting ≥50% stenoses by QCA decreased from

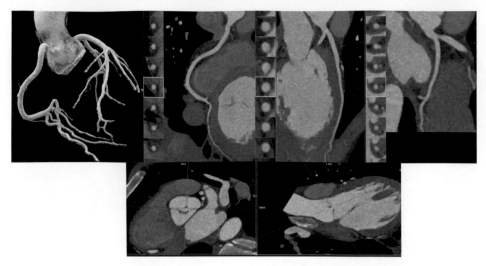

Figure 8.9 Negative predictive value. Coronary CTA is characterized by a very high negative predictive value. For example, in this patient with aortic insufficiency (lower left and right panels), coronary CTA 'ruled out' CAD prior to valve surgery.

99% on a patient level to 88% on a segment-based analysis and positive predictive value fell from 86% to 47%. Extensive data has accumulated demonstrating the prognostic information of CTA identified significant stenosis on future cardiovascular events.[109,110]

Based on these results, CTA is suitable for clinical situations in which the exclusion of significant proximal disease is required, specifically patients with non-acute symptoms and intermediate pretest probability, in particular if stress testing is not an option.

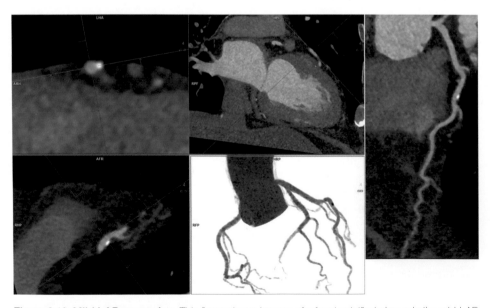

Figure 8.10 Mild LAD narrowing. This figure shows images of a focal calcified plaque in the mid-LAD with minimal luminal narrowing (<25%).

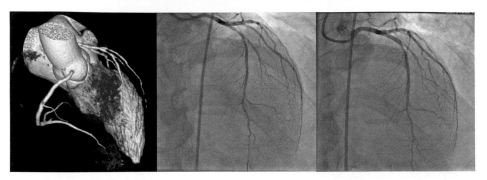

Figure 8.11 LAD stenosis (1). This figure shows VRI images of the CTA and images of the coronary angiogram of a patient with a significant lesion in the mid-LAD.

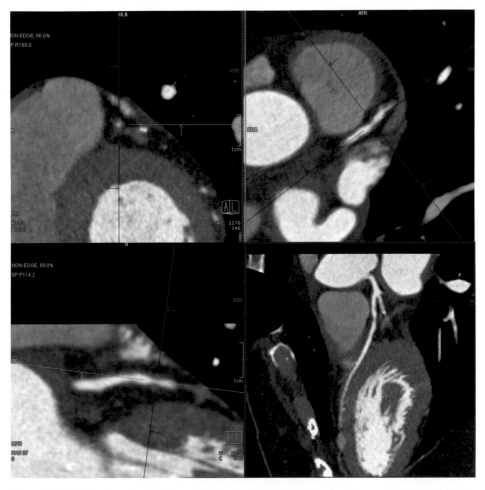

Figure 8.12 LAD stenosis (2). These MPR images again show the focal non-calcified lesion in the mid-LAD.

95

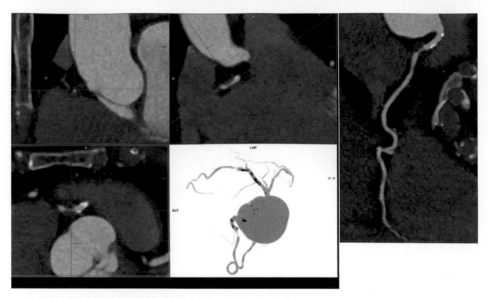

Figure 8.13 Significant proximal RCA lesion. This figure shows images of partially calcified plaque in the proximal RCA with a focal non-calcified plaque with significant luminal narrowing (>70%).

Coronary CTA allows assessment of bypass graft starts with identification of the native ostial and vessels, both for location and patency. A systematic approach for bypass graft identification starts with identification of the native coronary ostia and then searches the wall of the ascending aorta for evidence of patent occluded aorto-coronary

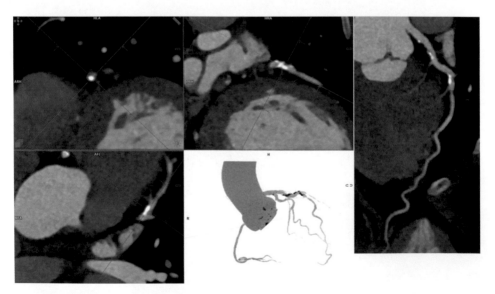

Figure 8.14 LAD same patient. The LAD in the same patient shows a densely calcific lesion in the proximal LAD. Precise assessment is limited by calcium 'blooming' artefact, but significant stenosis (>50%) is suspected.

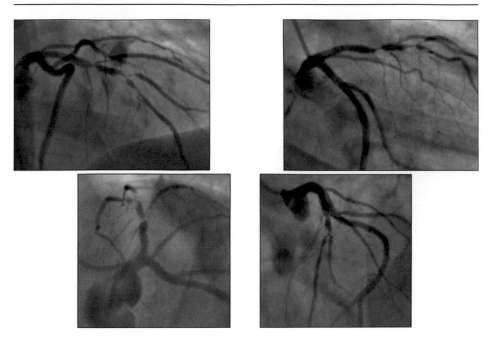

Figure 8.15 **Significant luminal stenosis (1), angiography.** This figure shows angiographic images from a patient with significant luminal stenoses of the left anterior descending coronary artery (LAD).

grafts. This is followed by identification of the left internal thoracic/right internal thoracic arteries (LITA/RITA) (**Figure 8.20**). Assessment of graft patency may be limited by surgical clips, but detailed reconstruction often allows assessment including of the distal anastomosis (**Figures 8.21** and **8.22**). Other findings, including stents and graft aneurysms, can be described (**Figures 8.23–8.26**). An important application is the assessment of graft position before repeating bypass surgery to avoid injury during surgery.[111]

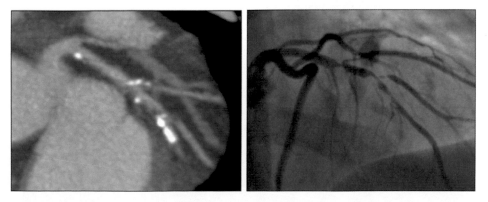

Figure 8.16 **Significant luminal stenosis (2), lesion characteristics.** Dense calcification of the plaque at the lesion site of the LAD is clearly shown on the MPR image, and precludes precise luminal assessment with CT. The coronary angiogram provides superior imaging of the luminal stenosis.

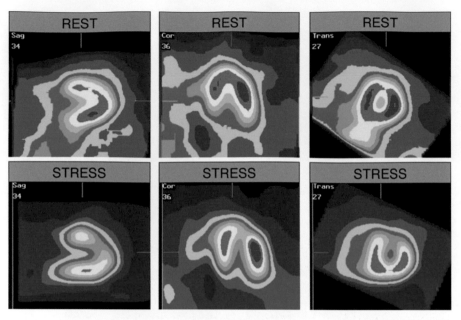

Figure 8.17 Significant luminal stenosis (3), ischemia. This figure shows corresponding images of the nuclear stress test. Apical ischemia, corresponding to the LAD lesions, is documented.

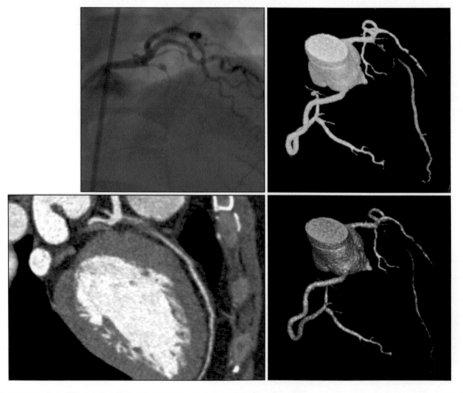

Figure 8.18 LAD occlusion (1). Images of a patient with chronic proximal LAD occlusion. The distal LAD fills via collaterals. The MPR image (left lower panel) shows the significant plaque burden at the lesion site, which is associated with expansive remodelling.

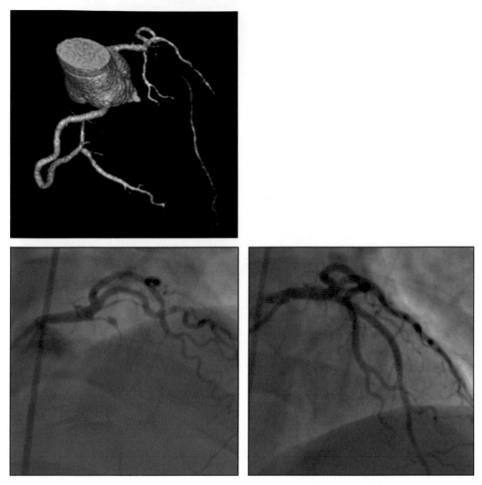

Figure 8.19 LAD occlusion (2), PCI. This figure shows pre- and post-interventional images of this patient with chronic proximal LAD occlusion. The proximal LAD lesions were stented.

Metal blooming artefact from the high-density metallic mesh of coronary stents frequently precludes confident detection and grading of in-stent restenosis with CT. However, differentiation between stent patency and occlusion and evaluation of stenosis at the leading or trailing ends of a stent are often possible (**Figures 8.27–8.29**).[112] Inferring stent patency from the presence of luminal enhancement distal to the stent is limited, because retrograde filling from collaterals cannot be differentiated by CT.

Other clinical indications for coronary CTA may include:

- Proximal coronary dissection (**Figure 8.30**). It is important to remember that assessment of coronary dissection in more distal vessel segments is unreliable with CT.[113,114]
- Pre-interventional assessment of lesion calcification and assessment of unclear left main coronary artery lesions (**Figures 8.31–8.35**).
- Non-stenotic forms of atherosclerotic disease including diffuse coronary ectasia and focal aneurysmal dilatation (**Figures 8.36** and **8.37**).

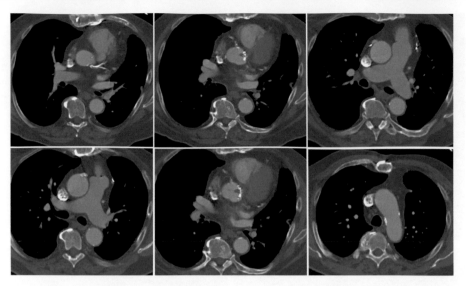

Figure 8.20 **Bypass graft assessment.** A systematic approach for bypass graft identification starts with identification of the native coronary ostia and then searches the wall of the ascending aorta for evidence of patent occluded aorto-coronary grafts. This is followed by identification of the left internal thoracic/right internal thoracic arteries (LITA/RITA)

- Non-atherosclerotic aneurysms (**Figures 8.38–8.41**)
- Coronary fistulas (**Figure 8.42**)
- Coronary anomalies are described in Chapter 13. As an example, a patient with ALCAPA is shown in **Figure 8.43**

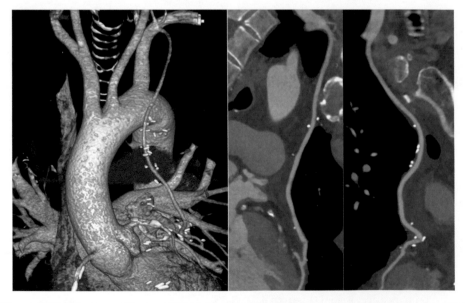

Figure 8.21 **Bypass graft assessment (1), distal anastomosis.** Detailed reconstruction often allows assessment including of the distal anastomosis, as shown for this LITA graft anastomosed to the mid-LAD.

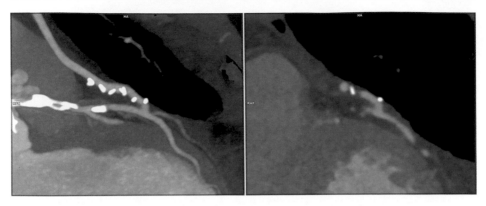

Figure 8.22 Bypass graft assessment (2), distal anastomosis. The distal anastomosis is shown in the images this figure.

8.1.2 Assessment of Hemodynamic Significance of Coronary Lesions

An optimized diagnostic approach to coronary artery disease combines assessment of lesion anatomy with evaluation of hemodynamic significance. Fractional flow reserve (CT-FFR), myocardial perfusion imaging, and transluminal attenuation gradient (TAG) are techniques that can be performed at the time of coronary CTA. CT-FFR describes dedicated, complex fluid dynamic calculations based on rest coronary anatomy.[115,116] The results are displayed

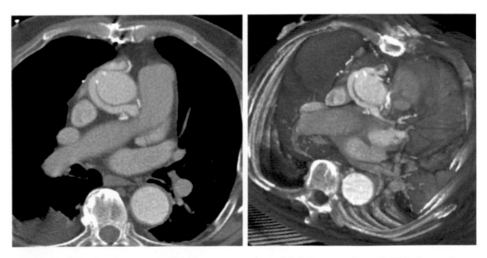

Figure 8.23 Re-implantation of coronary arteries with interposed graft. This figure shows images of a patient with remote history of aortic valve replacement with valved conduit and re-implantation of the coronary arteries into the mid-portion of the valved conduit of the ascending aorta. There is an interposed graft originating above the right coronary cusp and immediately bifurcating into two limbs (Cabrol interposition graft). One limb connects to the right coronary artery. There is a small aneurysmal dilatation at the anastomosis with the right coronary artery. The other limb takes a course behind the aorta and connects to the left main coronary artery. The graft and the proximal native coronary arteries are patent.

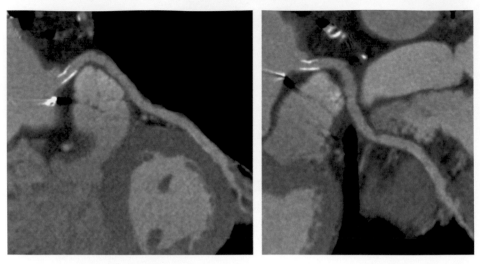

Figure 8.24 Stented bypass graft (1), stent patency. Because of their large size, stents in coronary bypass grafts can often be assessed for patency and severity of stenosis. The images in this figure show a patent stent in the ostial left main coronary artery.

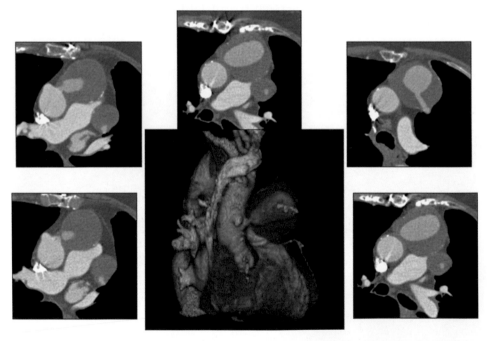

Figure 8.25 Bypass graft aneurysm (2), CT. There is a patent saphenous vein graft to the circumflex artery, which is aneurysmally dilated in its proximal segments. The aneurysmally dilated, partially thrombosed segment at the origin of the graft measures 6.9 cm in its largest diameter. The diameter of the contrast-filled lumen reaches 4.3 cm. There is a smaller aneurysmal dilatation measuring 3 cm, with normal luminal diameter (right upper panel). There is no evidence of luminal stenosis. There are additional stumps of aorto-coronary grafts seen in the ascending aorta.

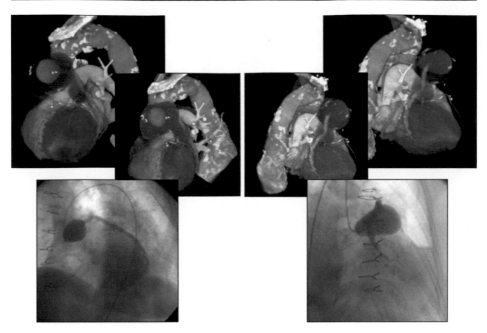

Figure 8.26 **Bypass graft aneurysm, angiography and CT.** The comparison between angiographic and CT images demonstrates the aneurysmally dilated segments in the proximal segments of the graft. The angiogram shows the perfused lumen, while the CT also shows the thrombus-filled aneurysm sac, surrounding the contrast-filled lumen.

in colour maps of the coronary tree reflecting hemodynamic significance of focal lesions (**Figure 8.44**). Perfusion imaging acquires myocardial perfusion at rest and pharmacological stress (vasodilator).[117–119] The technique allows construction of time-attenuation curves, which describe the delivery of contrast into the myocardium, and its subsequent washout over time (**Figures 8.45–8.47**). TAG described the change in luminal attenuation along a segment of the coronary arteries.[120]

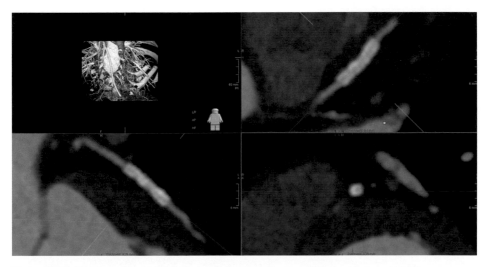

Figure 8.27 **Coronary stents.** This figure shows images of a patent stent in the mid-LAD.

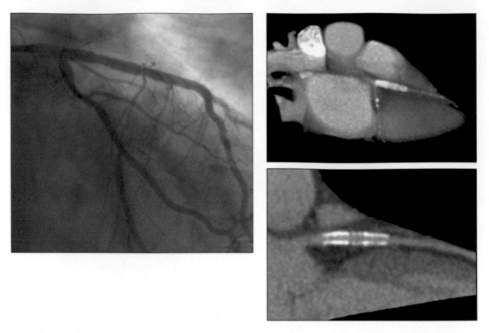

Figure 8.28 Coronary stent. This figure shows images of a patient that underwent percutaneous coronary intervention with placement of overlapping stent in the proximal LAD. The post-interventional angiogram and corresponding CT images are shown. Precise assessment of luminal dimensions inside the stents is limited with CT secondary to the blooming artefact of the stent struts.

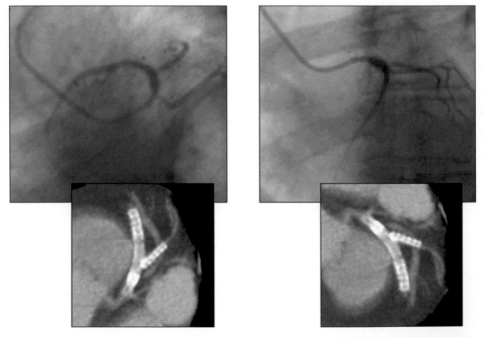

Figure 8.29 Coronary stent, diagonal branch. This figure shows pre-interventional angiographic and CT images of a patient with in-stent restenosis of a previous stent deployed in the first diagonal branch of the LAD. There are additional patent stents in the proximal LAD. Because of the small size of the stent, the stenotic lumen cannot be reliably assessed with CT.

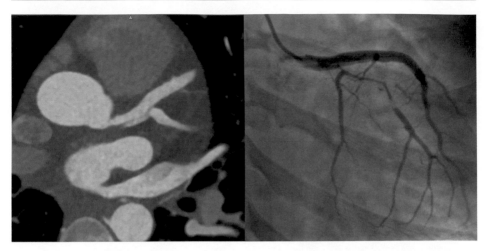

Figure 8.30 Left main coronary dissection. The figure in the left panel shows evidence of coronary dissection in the left main coronary artery. The corresponding angiogram is shown in the right panel.

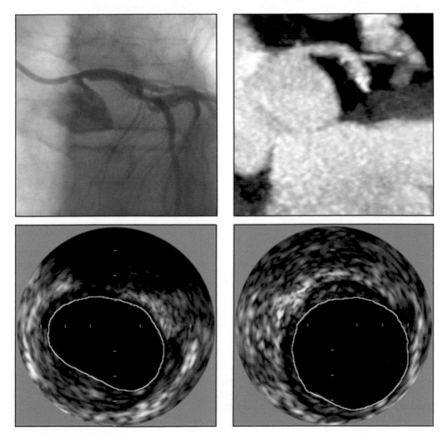

Figure 8.31 Left main disease. A patient with equivocal stress test results and suspected atherosclerotic disease of the left main coronary artery was referred for further evaluation. The cardiac CT (right upper panel) shows ostial narrowing with suspected atherosclerotic plaque accumulation. Cardiac catheterization (left upper panel) confirmed ostial stenosis of the left main coronary artery. IVUS showed ostial atherosclerotic plaque with mild, 30% cross-sectional narrowing. Aggressive risk factor modification was instituted.

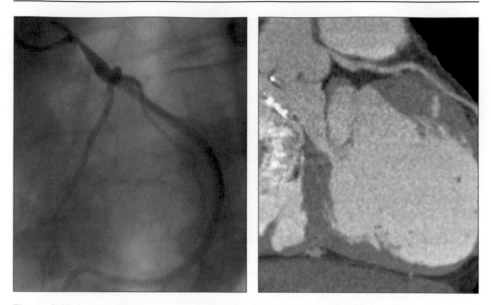

Figure 8.32 Left main compression and VSD (1). These images show a patient with a remote history of VSD repair, who presented with shortness of breath. A cardiac catheterization showed ostial stenosis of the left main coronary artery. Based on the angiographic appearance, external compression of the left main coronary artery was suspected. The patient was referred for CTA. This figure shows the comparison between angiographic and VRI CT images. The ostial narrowing of the left main coronary artery (LM) is seen in both images. The corresponding MPR image (right panel) again demonstrates the ostial narrowing. However, there is no associated atherosclerotic plaque accumulation of the left main. The pulmonary artery is prominent and appears to compress the left main coronary artery.

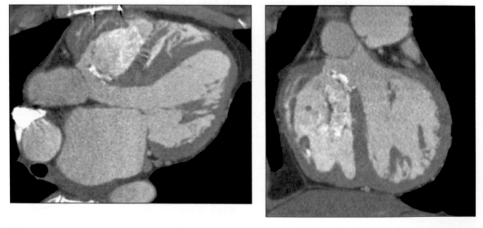

Figure 8.33 Left main compression, VSD repair (2). This figure demonstrates the cause of the dilated pulmonary artery. It shows evidence of remote repair of a VSD in the left ventricular outflow tract with surgical material. However, there is residual VSD with suspected shunting to the right ventricle and subsequent volume overload. This causes pulmonary artery dilatation and subsequent left main compression.

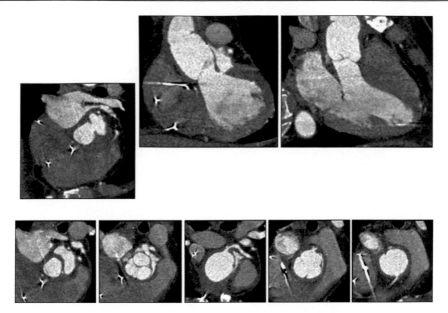

Figure 8.34 **Left-ventricular (LV) outflow tract pseudoaneurysm causing coronary compression (1).** A patient presented with atypical chest pain and history of aortic valve replacement with a homograft. A cardiac catheterization demonstrated systolic compression of the left main and left anterior descending coronary artery. The CT images show evidence of replacement of the ascending aorta. There is wall thickening of the homograft extending into the proximal segments of the re-implanted coronary arteries compatible with inflammatory material. A pseudoaneurysm originates from the anterior left aspect of the left ventricular outflow tract below the aortic valve level. The cavity lies on the left side of the homograft and extends up to the level of the left main coronary artery ostium. The dimensions of the pseudoaneurysm are 2.5 × 3 × 3.5 cm in diastole and 3.6 × 4.0 × 3.8 cm in systole.

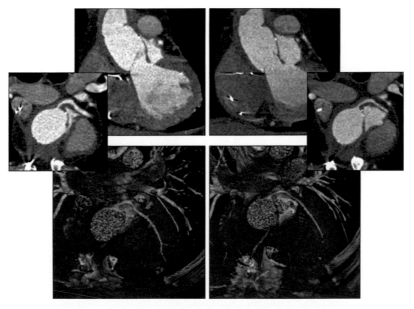

Figure 8.35 **LV outflow tract pseudoaneurysm causing coronary compression (2).** The pseudoaneurysm appears to be the cause of the systolic coronary compression of the left main coronary artery and proximal LAD coronary artery, which are draped around the cavity.

107

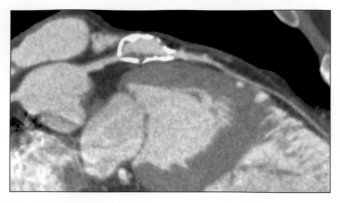

Figure 8.36 Left anterior descending coronary aneurysm. This figure shows a focal aneurysm of the proximal LAD with extensive calcification of the aneurysm wall. MPR image is showing the calcified wall of the aneurysm and the small amount of adherent wall thrombus inside the aneurysm.

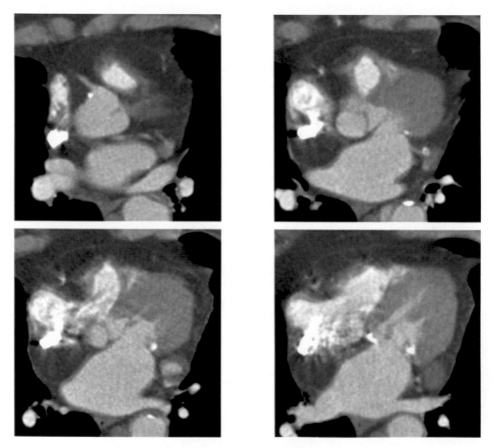

Figure 8.37 Left circumflex coronary aneurysm. An example of a focal aneurysm of the left circumflex coronary artery (LCX) is shown in these four axial images (cranial to caudal). There is calcification of the LCX proximal to the aneurysm and a moderate amount of adherent wall thrombus inside the aneurysm.

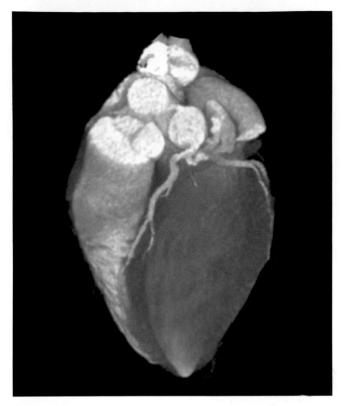

Figure 8.38 Left main coronary aneurysm. Non-atherosclerotic aneurysmal disease is also seen with inflammatory diseases. This figure shows a large left main coronary artery aneurysm in a patient with a history of Kawasaki disease.

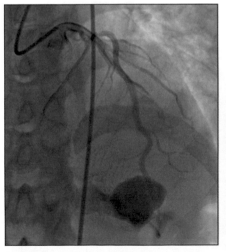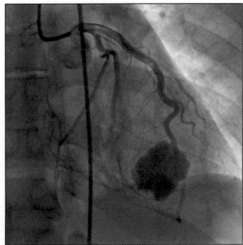

Figure 8.39 LAD inflammatory aneurysm, angiogram (1). Images of a patient with a suspected inflammatory coronary aneurysm. The patient presented with acute coronary syndrome. Cardiac catheterization demonstrated a contrast-filled structure in the distal LAD distribution, measuring about 3 cm. There appears to be a small communication with the right ventricle, with a small amount of contrast seen as it is ejected through the RV and RV outflow tract in the cineangiogram.

109

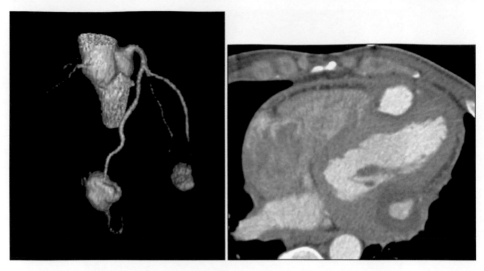

Figure 8.40 LAD inflammatory aneurysm, CT (2). A cardiac CTA clearly demonstrates the aneurysms of the LAD and LCX. A rim of thrombus is seen in the LAD aneurysm. CT defined the entry and exit points of the LAD and LCX into the aneurysm.

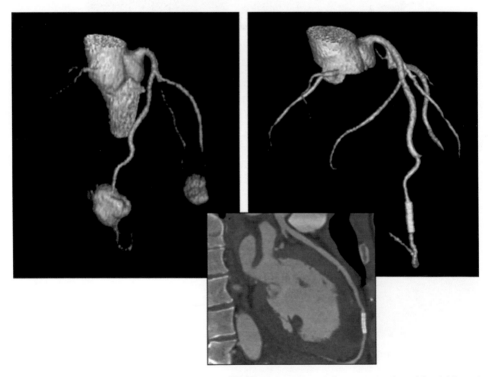

Figure 8.41 LAD inflammatory aneurysm, CT (3). The patient underwent stenting of the LAD and LCX, with exclusion of the aneurysms. This figure shows corresponding CT images before (left panel) and after (right panel) PCI.

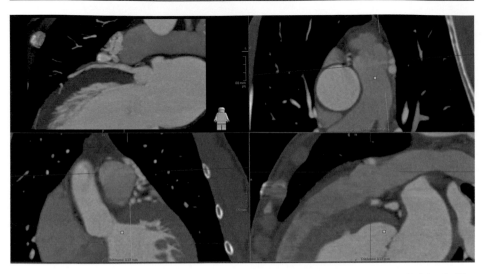

Figure 8.42 LAD to PA fistula. This figure shows a LAD coronary to pulmonary artery (PA) fistula. The left upper panel shows the origin of the fistula from the proximal LAD, continuing in a tortuous vessel adjacent to the central PA. The left lower panel appears to show a small jet at the site of communication with the PA.

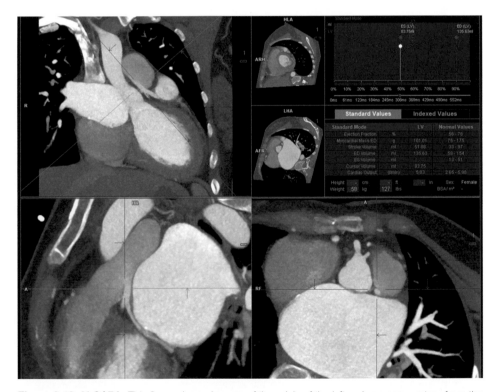

Figure 8.43 ALCAPA. This figure shows images of the origin of the left main coronary artery from the central PA. The higher contrast enhancement in the coronary artery relative to the PA is evidence of retrograde drainage from the left main into the PA.

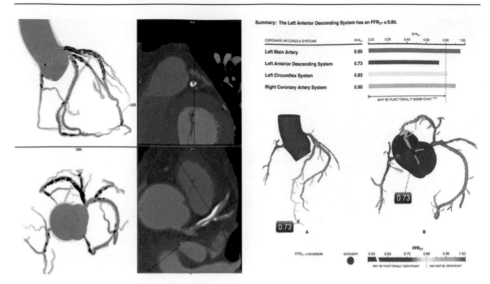

Figure 8.44 CT-FFR. CT-FFR describes dedicated, complex fluid dynamic calculations based on rest coronary anatomy. The results are displayed in colour maps of the coronary tree reflecting hemodynamic significance of focal lesions.

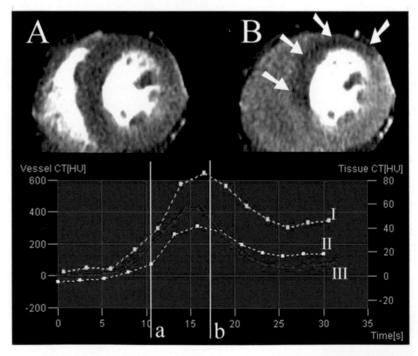

Figure 8.45 Dynamic CT MPI TACs and snapshot images. The graph shows typical time-attenuation curves (TACs) acquired with dynamic computed tomography (CT) myocardial perfusion imaging (MPI), and two snapshot images of the same mid-ventricular slice, corresponding to different time points of the CT MPI scan. The yellow curve (I) in the graph represents the TAC in normal tissue, the grey curve (II) that of infarcted area. The red curve (III) is the TAC of the ascending aorta. Image (A) was taken at the time point indicated by line (a) in the graph. Image (B) was taken 6 seconds later, as indicated by line (b). The variation between the images emphasizes the difficulty of timing a static scan to robustly assess the extent of a perfusion defect. HU = Hounsfield unit.

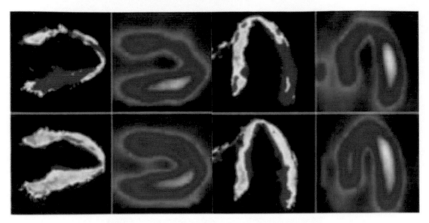

Figure 8.46 Display of CT myocardial perfusion images. Display of CT myocardial perfusion images in the short-axis, vertical and horizontal long-axis views. In each view, the stress image is in the upper row and the rest image below. The corresponding nuclear perfusion image is displayed side by side.

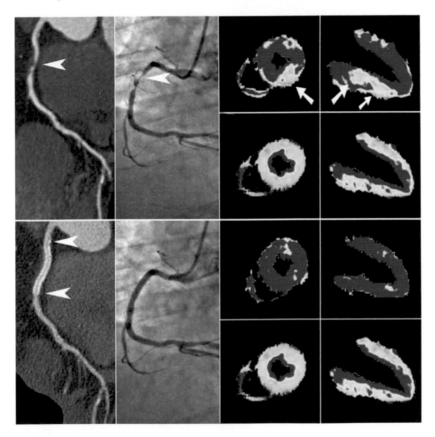

Figure 8.47 Resolution of perfusion defect after PCI. CT angiogram of the mid-RCA showing 95% stenosis (top row, before stent, arrowheads), with correlation of invasive angiography, and the presence of a reversible defect (green) of the inferolateral wall (arrows) shown on stress (top) and rest (bottom) CTMPI. After stent (bottom row), the CT angiogram of mid-RCA shows the patent stent (arrowheads), with correlation of invasive angiography. There is resolution of the reversible defect of the inferolateral wall on stress (top), compared with the initial rest scan (bottom) as a reference.

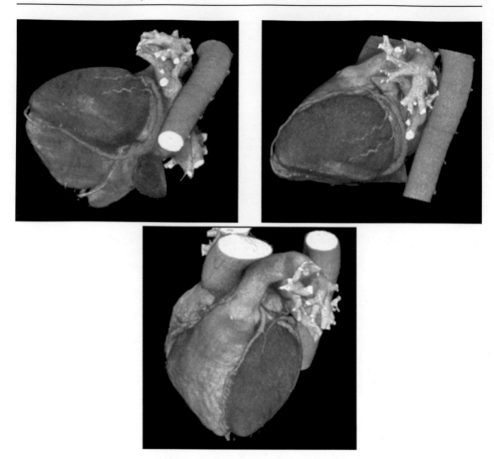

Figure 8.48 Normal coronary sinus/coronary vein anatomy. In this figure, normal vein anatomy is shown. The great cardiac vein runs parallel to the proximal LAD (lower panel), then follows the LCX into the atrioventricular groove (right upper panel), and drains into the right atrium as the coronary sinus (left upper panel).

8.1.3 Coronary Veins and Coronary Sinus

Because of the peripheral intravenous rather than selective arterial contrast injection, the coronary sinus and coronary veins are typically slightly contrast-enhanced on CT images. The course of coronary veins is parallel to the course of the coronary arteries. Therefore, if venous enhancement is more pronounced (e.g. in more venous phase images), the veins can be mistaken for coronary arteries. If the venous structures are the primary focus of the examination, contrast timing is adjusted (**Figures 8.48–8.50**). Clinical indications include assessment of the coronary sinus anatomy/coronary veins for the placement of biventricular pacer leads or studies performed prior to lead extraction.[121,122]

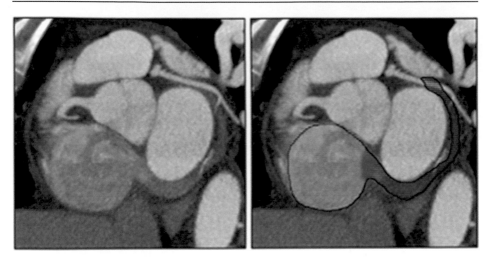

Figure 8.49 Coronary sinus. In this figure, the right atrium (yellow) and coronary sinus (red) is illustrated. The coronary sinus has several branches. The branch shown in this image continues along the left AV groove to the anterior interventricular groove.

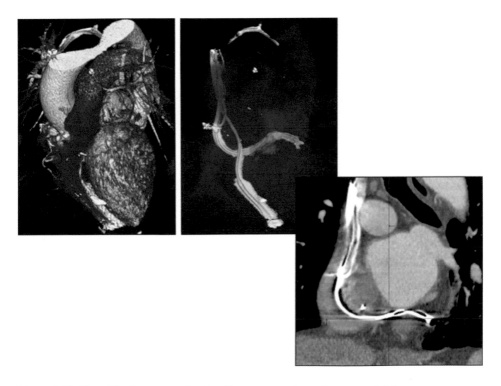

Figure 8.50 Biventricular pacemaker lead in coronary sinus. Assessment of the coronary venous anatomy is performed prior to placement of biventricular pacer leads. In this figure, pacer leads of a biventricular pacing lead are visible in the right ventricle and coronary sinus.

Pulmonary Vascular Disease

9.1 Pulmonary Artery

Compared with ventilation–perfusion (VQ) scans, contrast-enhanced CT has a high sensitivity and specificity for the diagnosis of pulmonary embolism (main through segmental arteries) (**Figure 9.1**).[123] The advantages of CT are the speed and the wide availability in emergency departments. The CT scan allows direct visualization of the thrombus, and simultaneous assessment of the lung parenchyma and size of the cardiac chambers (e.g. right ventricular enlargement). On the other hand, CT does not provide an assessment of lung ventilation or perfusion (VQ scan) or right ventricular function (echocardiography, MRI). Pulmonary CT angiography can occasionally show other findings, including PA pseudoaneurysms (**Figure 9.2**).

9.2 Pulmonary Veins

In congenital heart disease, pulmonary vein anatomy is relevant in the assessment of abnormal venous return (see Chapter 11). In the context of electrophysiology, pulmonary vein anatomy is relevant for treatment planning and assessment of complications of percutaneous ablation procedures at the pulmonary vein ostia for chronic atrial fibrillation. Imaging of the pulmonary veins before the procedure for 3-D guidance and more frequently after the procedure for diagnosis and surveillance of pulmonary vein stenosis is now commonly performed.[124] Post-interventional complications include wall thickening and luminal stenosis (**Figures 9.3–9.7**). CT is sensitive in identifying and grading stenosis, but limited in differentiating subtotal and total venous occlusion. An important advantage of CT is the ability to visualize inflammatory changes associated with the development of vein stenosis, including wall thickening at the vein ostia and mediastinal lymph node enlargement. Other imaging modalities including echocardiography and MRI can reliably image the pulmonary veins.[125] If severe pulmonary vein stenosis requires angioplasty and stenting, pre-procedural planning and post-procedural assessment of stent position and patency can reliably be performed with CT (**Figures 9.8** and **9.9**).

Other infrequent complications of ablation include LA-esophageal fistulas (**Figure 9.10**).

As described in Chapter 4, CT allows assessment of the left atrium and left atrial appendage and identification of thrombus and slow flow (**Figures 4.27** and **9.11**). The left atrial appendage is further assessment prior to and following placement of LAA occluding devices (**Figure 9.12**).[126,127]

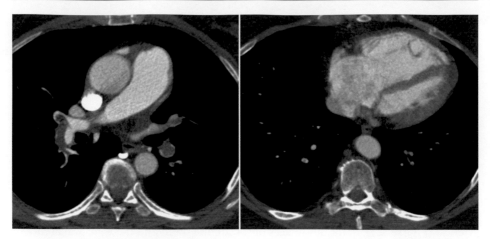

Figure 9.1 Pulmonary embolism. This figure shows images of a bilateral central-filling defect of the pulmonary arteries, consistent with acute PE. There is associated enlargement of the right ventricle.

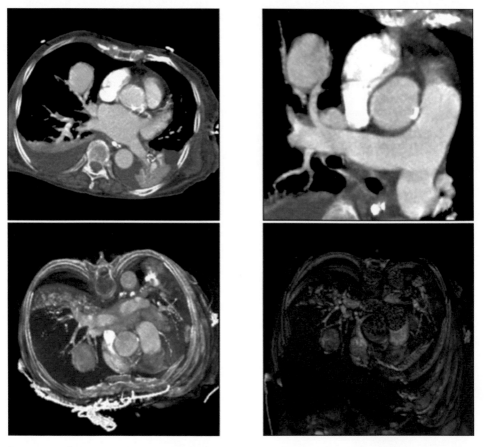

Figure 9.2 Pulmonary artery pseudoaneurysm. This figure shows images of a patient with a pseudoaneurysm following the placement of a pulmonary artery catheter. The pseudoaneurysm arises from the right middle lobe pulmonary artery, and measures approximately 4.0 × 3.3 cm.

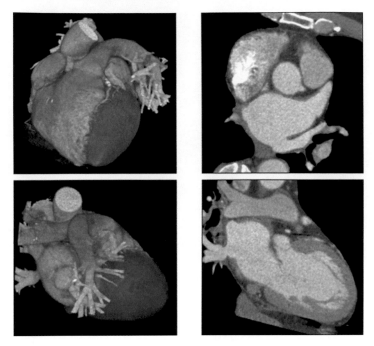

Figure 9.3 Pulmonary vein stenosis (1). Images taken 3 months after pulmonary vein isolation (PVI). The left atrium and left atrial appendage show no evidence of thrombus (right upper panel). There is thickening of the vessel wall at the right inferior pulmonary vein ostium, with about 40% luminal stenosis (right lower panel).

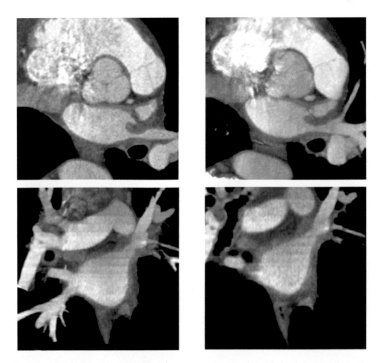

Figure 9.4 Pulmonary vein stenosis (2). More severe narrowing of the left superior vein ostium after ablation is shown in figure. Note the location of the left atrial appendage anterior to the left superior vein ostium.

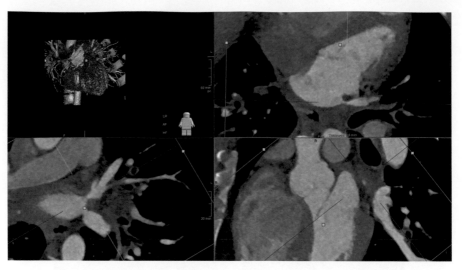

Figure 9.5 Pulmonary vein stenosis (3). Severe stenosis of the left superior vein ostium after pulmonary vein ablation is shown in this figure.

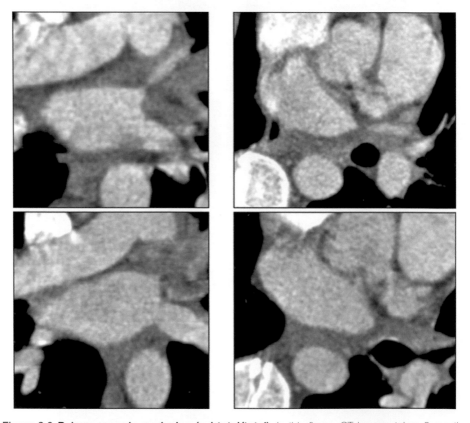

Figure 9.6 Pulmonary vein occlusion (subtotal/total). In this figure, CT images taken 3 months (upper panels) and 6 months (lower panels) after vein ablation are shown. There is an increase in stenosis of the pulmonary vein ostia with total/subtotal occlusion of the left superior vein ostium. However, CT is limited in differentiating subtotal and total occlusion, which can be assessed with pulmonary angiography.

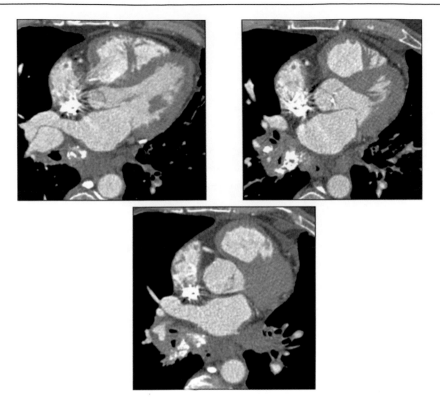

Figure 9.7 Fibrosing mediastinitis with pulmonary vein occlusion. This figure shows images of a patient with fibrosing mediastinitis. There is partially calcified soft tissue in the mediastinum surrounding the left atrium. Only the right superior vein is patent. The other veins are occluded.

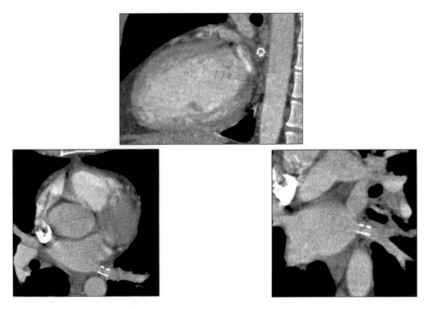

Figure 9.8 Pulmonary vein stent (1). This figure shows images of a patent stent in left inferior pulmonary vein ostium.

121

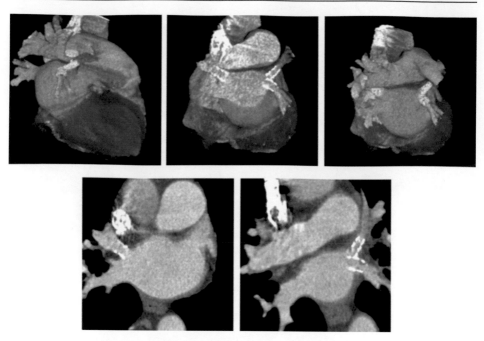

Figure 9.9 Pulmonary vein stent (2). This figure shows patent stents of the right superior, left superior, and left inferior veins. Both left-sided stents demonstrate small amounts of soft tissue lining the stent lumen. However, assessment of in-stent thrombosis or neointimal tissue inside the stents is limited with CT.

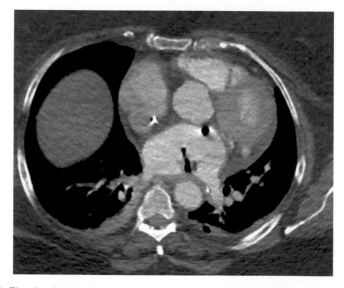

Figure 9.10 Fistula between LA and esophagus. This figure shows evidence of a LA-esophageal fistula after ablation. Air is seen in the left atrium, with high risk of symptomatic air embolization.

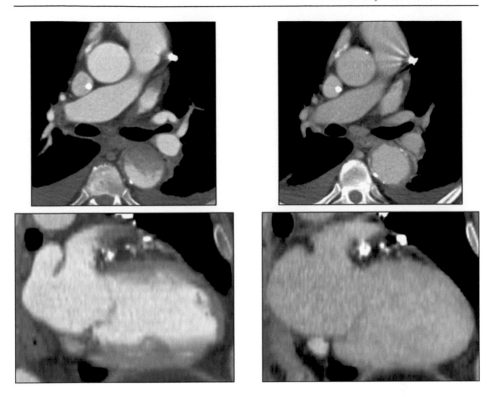

Figure 9.11 Thrombus versus slow flow. CT allows to differentiate thrombus left atrial appendage thrombus from slow flow. This figure shows filling defects in the LAA in the images obtained immediately after contrast administration (left panels, arterial phase). The filling defects disappear in delayed acquired images (right panels, venous phase), consistent with slow flow.

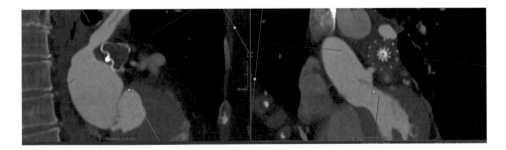

Figure 9.12 Watchman. This figure shows images after LAA occluding device placement (Watchman). The device is well seated without evidence of residual flow.

10

Aortic Disease

10.1 Aortic Disease

CT is the preferred imaging modality for a wide range of aortic pathology, including acute aortic syndromes (AAS) (aortic dissection and its variants, including trauma), inflammatory aortic disease, as well as elective imaging in the context of suspected aortic enlargement, surgical or endovascular treatment planning, surveillance, and follow-up.[128,129] Contrast enhancement is crucial for a majority of indications to differentiate the lumen and the vessel wall. However, non-contrast imaging of the aorta allows precise measurements of dimensions. Diagnostic alternatives include MRI and echocardiography (in particular TEE).

Modern multidetector scanners allow scanning of the entire thoracic and abdominal aorta in one breath-hold with or without ECG synchronization of the thoracic segments. ECG synchronization is achieved with standard retrospective-gated or prospective-triggered acquisition techniques, and is important for indications focused on the aortic root and ascending aorta in order to reduce cardiac motion artefacts transmitted to the aortic root (**Figure 10.1**).[130,131] However, modern scanners with larger number of detectors and faster rotation time frequently provide relatively motionless imaging even with non–ECG-synchronized acquisition. Non–ECG-synchronized/non-gated acquisitions of the chest, abdomen, and pelvis have the advantage of providing continuous data sets with homogeneous arterial enhancement of entire aorta including the arch and visceral branch vessels, and is therefore better suited for indications focused on the descending thoracoabdominal aorta including endovascular stent planning.

10.1.1 Acute Aortic Syndromes

CT imaging plays a critical role in the diagnosis and management of AAS.[132] Acute aortic syndrome is a clinical term describing an acute aortic pain syndrome associated with acute, life-threatening aortic diseases (in analogy to the term 'acute coronary syndrome'), and encompasses several different entities.[133] Classic aortic dissection describes a splitting or separation of the aortic wall within the media layer of the aorta. The pathological substrate that predisposes the aorta for dissection is an abnormal media layer, which is traditionally described as 'cystic medianecrosis.'[134] Medial degeneration can be caused by several entities, including congenital and genetic disorders (Marfan syndrome, Ehlers Danlos Type IV, aortitis), but is most commonly associated with severe, long-standing hypertension.

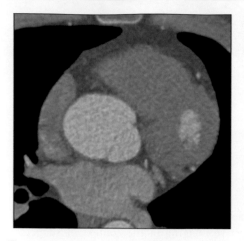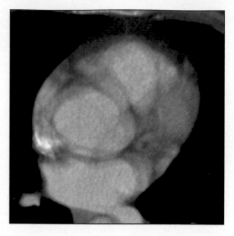

Figure 10.1 Motion artefact aortic root. Because of the rapid motion of the heart and the relatively long acquisition window of CT, blurring of the image occurs, in particular if the acquisition window is not synchronized to the cardiac cycle. In this image of a non-gated CT scan, image artefact at the aortic root is seen (right panel), which could be mistaken for a dissection flap. However, the symmetry with linear structure on both sides of the aortic root is more typical for motion artefact. The left panel shows the same images with an ECG-synchronized acquisition.

10.1.1.1 Morphologic classification

Anatomic manifestations of acute aortic dissection are classified in distinct morphologic classes[128]:

- *Class I* – Classic aortic dissection: characterized by a primary intimal tear, separation within the media with a true and false lumen divided by a 'flap,' and an exit- or re-entry tear. (**Figures 10.2–10.4**).
- *Class II* – Intramural hematoma (IMH): describes a variant of aortic dissection where the space within the diseased aortic media layer is filled with clotted blood rather than a flow channel ('false lumen') (**Figure 10.5**). High-quality CT scans occasionally allow to identify intimal tears, which are more frequently found during surgery or autopsy.
- *Class III* – Also called 'limited dissection' or 'focal intimal tears': describes localized confined intimal tears without extensive undermining of the intima or flap formation.[135,136] These are often seen with Marfan syndrome and can rupture or cause tamponade. The typical appearance is of a small outpouching of the aortic wall (**Figures 10.6** and **10.7**).
- *Class IV* – Penetrating atherosclerotic ulcers with localized dissections or wall hematomas: often with calcium at the base of a mushroom-shaped area of extraluminal contrast (**Figure 10.8**).
- *Class V* – Iatrogenic or posttraumatic dissection (**Figure 10.9**).

10.1.1.2 Location and extent

The anatomic extent and location of the dissection process have critical implications on treatment decisions. The traditional anatomic classifications for aortic dissection are the 1965 DeBakey classification, and the 1970 Stanford classification.[137,138] Similar to the DeBakey system, more recent classifications are based on the location of the primary

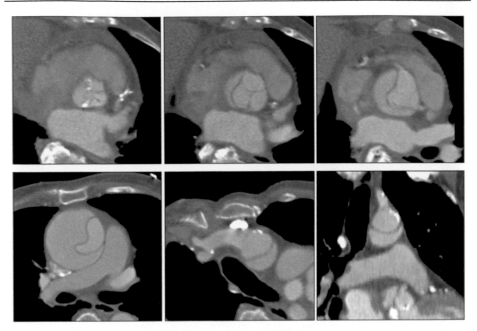

Figure 10.2 Type A aortic dissection (1) – Class I. The figure shows a type A dissection. The dissection flap originates in the aortic root (upper panels) and extends throughout the ascending thoracic aorta and aortic arch (lower panel). In the dilated mid-ascending aorta (lower left panel) the smaller true lumen is surrounded by the larger false lumen.

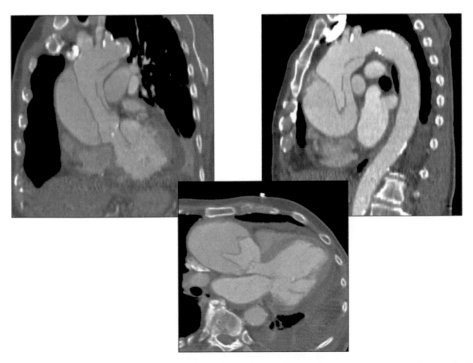

Figure 10.3 Type A aortic dissection (2) – Class I. In the same patient, the corresponding sagittal reconstructions show the extent of the dissection in the ascending aorta and aortic arch.

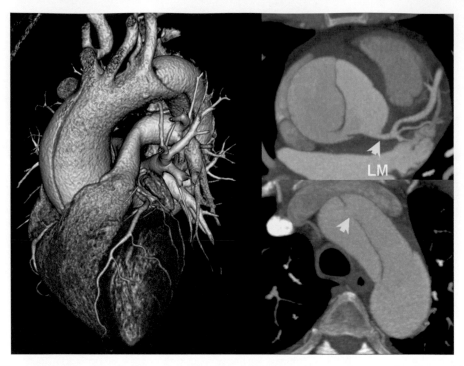

Figure 10.4 Type A aortic dissection (3) – Class I. This figure shows a volume-rendered image (left panel) and MRP images (right panels) of a patient with acute type A aortic dissection. The right upper panel defines the origin of the left main (LM) from the true lumen and shows the proximal entry tear. The right lower image shows a re-entry tear at the level of the aortic arch.

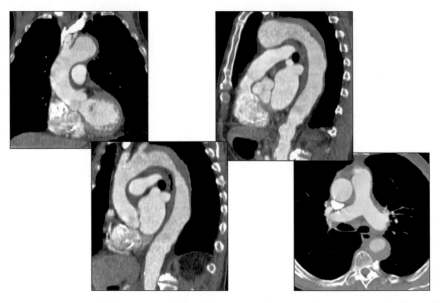

Figure 10.5 Intramural hematoma: Aortic dissection – Class II. The images in this figure show an intramural hematoma of the descending thoracic aorta. There is wall thickening of the isthmus and descending thoracic aorta (right upper panel). The cross-sectional image shows the crescentic shape of the intramural hematoma in the mid-descending aorta (right lower panel).

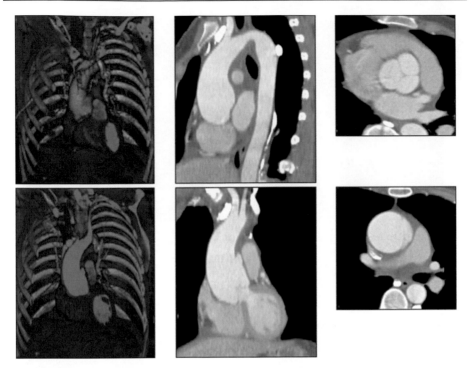

Figure 10.6 Acute penetrating ulceration/focal dissection: Aortic dissection (1) – Class II. This figure shows a focal penetrating ulceration/focal intimal tear in the proximal ascending aorta, associated with the clinical presentation of an acute aortic syndrome. Careful review of the axial images demonstrated evidence of mediastinal blood products, consistent with aortic leakage.

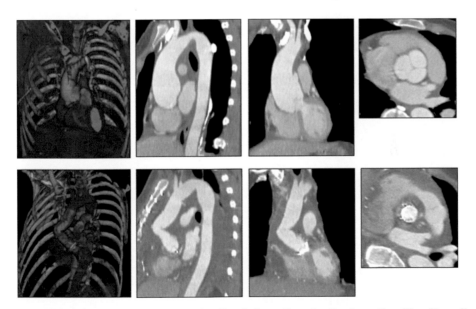

Figure 10.7 Acute penetrating ulceration/focal dissection: Aortic dissection (2) – Class II. The patient underwent urgent replacement of the ascending thoracic aorta with a composite graft. The mechanical aortic valve prosthesis and the grafts of the ascending aorta are seen in the postoperative images (lower panels).

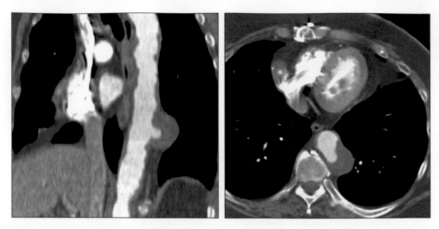

Figure 10.8 Penetrating ulceration. Penetrating ulcerations can be found in the context of acute and chronic aortic conditions. Penetrating atherosclerotic ulcers with localized dissections or wall hematomas are classified as Class IV dissection processes. This figure shows a focal, relatively large penetrating ulceration in the diffusely diseased retrocardiac descending thoracic aorta. Maximum diameter of the aorta at the level of the ulceration is 3.0 × 5.6 cm. The inhomogeneous Hounsfield units of the wall may be consistent with wall hematoma.

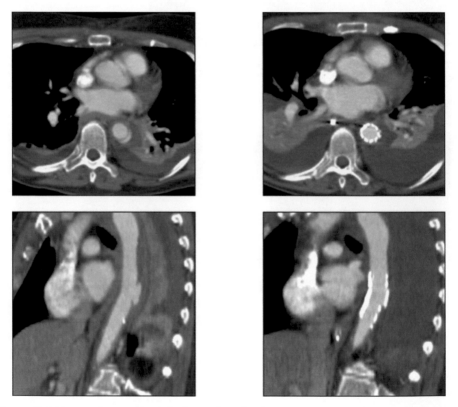

Figure 10.9 Traumatic type B aortic dissection. This figure shows images of a patient after recent motor vehicle accident. The left panels show axial (left upper panel) and sagittal (left lower panel) images of the descending aorta with a focal dissection. There are blood products in the adjacent mediastinum and layering of blood in the pleural effusion. The right panels show the corresponding images after treatment with an endovascular stent graft.

intimal tear.[139] The terms type A and type B are also used to describe the location of aortic IMH or penetrating ulcers.

10.1.1.3 Diagnostic considerations

MDCT is highly diagnostic for the identification of AAS. In the diagnostic assessment of acute aortic disorders, motionless assessment of the aortic root and ascending aorta is critical for management decisions. However, the cardiac pulsation is transmitted to the aortic root and ascending aorta, and often causes significant motion artefact (**Figure 10.1**). ECG-synchronized acquisition protocols substantially reduce motion artefact and should be used if detailed assessment of the aortic root and ascending aorta is required.

While Class I dissections with visible dissection flap are seldom missed, knowledge about the appearance of IMH is critical for its identification (**Figures 10.5** and **10.10**).[140]

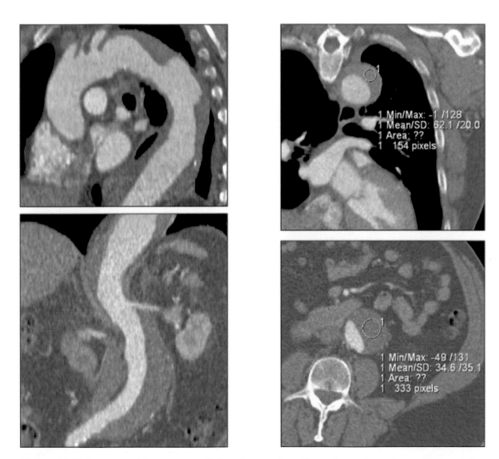

Figure 10.10 Intramural hematoma of the descending thoracic aorta and aneurysm of the abdominal aorta. This figure shows an intramural hematoma of the descending thoracic aorta with enlargement of the involved aortic segments (upper panels). Maximum diameter in the retrocardiac descending aorta is 6.3 cm. There is a large area of communication/breakdown between the lumen and the hematoma in the proximal descending aorta. The intramural hematoma ends in the suprarenal aorta. There is an additional infrarenal abdominal aortic aneurysm with maximum diameter of 5.1 cm (lower panels). The differences in Hounsfield units help to differentiate the two entities.

In the acute phase, the blood products in the wall have high Hounsfield units (HU) (in the range of 60–70), which is higher than unenhanced blood in the aortic lumen. Therefore, an IMH is easily identified on a non–contrast-enhanced scan as a rim of high signal (**Figures 10.10** and **10.11**). In the subacute phase, the HU decreases (**Figure 10.11**). An interesting aspect of IMH is its temporal change. Patterns of regression, evolution in Class I dissection, development of ulcer-like projections, and intramural blood pools are described (**Figures 10.12–10.15**).[141–143] It is important to differentiate blood product in the aortic wall (IMH) from structures adjacent to the aortic wall, including pericardial fluid in the folds adjacent to the ascending aorta, atelectasis adjacent to the descending aorta, and lung masses (**Figures 10.16–10.18**).

Acute penetrating ulcerations with localized dissections or wall hematomas can be identified with CT (**Figures 10.8** and **10.19**). Similarly, in patients presenting with painful or leaking degenerative aneurysms, CT is critical in presence of location of the aneurysm and

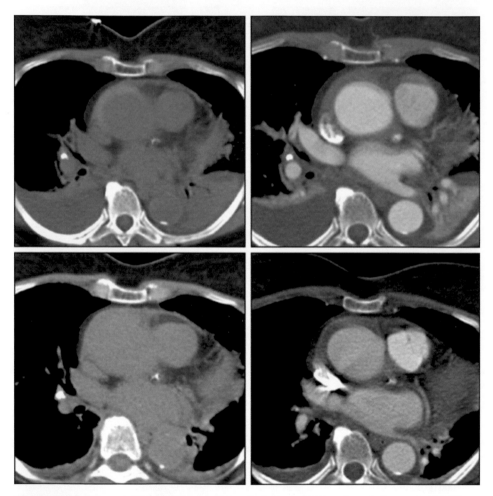

Figure 10.11 Intramural hematoma – Increased Hounsfield units of the wall. This figure demonstrates the increased HU of an acute IMH (left upper panel). After 1 week, the HU has decreased (left lower panel).

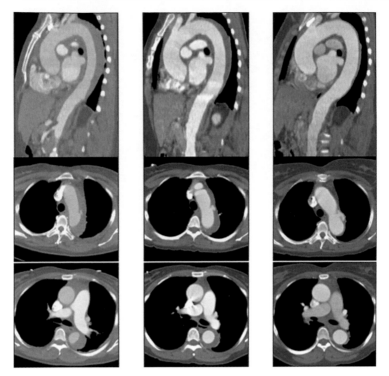

Figure 10.12 Resolving intramural hematoma. This figure shows a chronic intramural hematoma with evidence of partial resolution. The upper (sagittal) and lower (axial) panels show significant wall thickening at baseline (left panel) and gradual resolution over the next 6 months (3 months – middle panel and 6 months – right panel). However, there is development of a focal pseudoaneurysm/ulcer-like projection at the aortic isthmus (middle panels), which was subsequently treated with an endovascular stent graft.

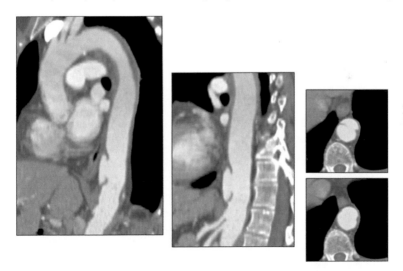

Figure 10.13 Intramural hematoma – Ulcer-like projection. This figure shows a chronic intramural hematoma of the descending thoracic aorta. Wall thickening of the isthmus and upper descending thoracic aorta is consistent with residuals of an intramural hematoma. In the descending thoracic aorta, there is an area of intimal disruption associated with mild bulging of the aorta (3.9 cm). The appearance is that of a penetrating ulceration.

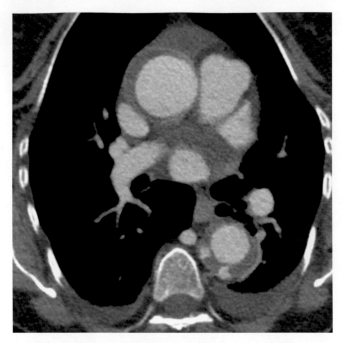

Figure 10.14 Intramural hematoma – Intramural bloodpool. This figure shows two intramural bloodpools in the medial aspect of the descending thoracic aorta; related to the intercostal arteries.

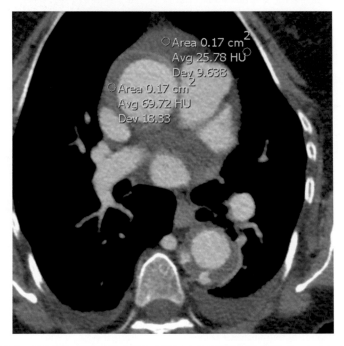

Figure 10.15 Intramural hematoma and fluid in pericardial fold. This figure shows an intramural hematoma of the ascending aorta and adjacent simple fluid in the pericardial fold. The normal pericardium extends up along parts of the ascending aorta and fluid in the pericardial fold is sometimes more difficult to differentiate from wall changes of an IMH than in this example.

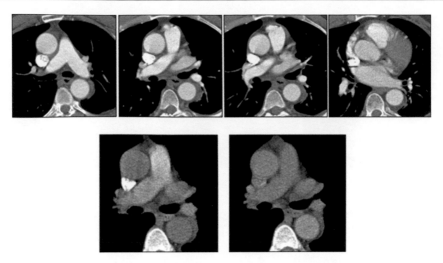

Figure 10.16 Intramural hematoma, differential diagnosis (1). The images in this figure show a small rim of atelectasis of the lung adjacent to descending thoracic aorta, which mimics the crescentic appearance of an intramural hematoma. The upper panels show different axial slices at the level around the bifurcation of the pulmonary arteries. The lower images show images early and late during injection of the contrast bolus.

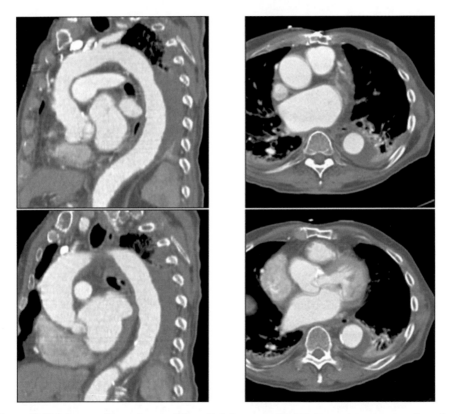

Figure 10.17 Intramural hematoma, differential diagnosis (2). This figure shows images of a patient with bilateral small to moderate-size pleural effusions. In the descending thoracic aorta, the fluid lies adjacent to the aorta and on some images has an appearance similar to an aneurysm or intramural hematoma (upper panels). However, close observation demonstrates that aortic wall and fluid are separate (lower panels).

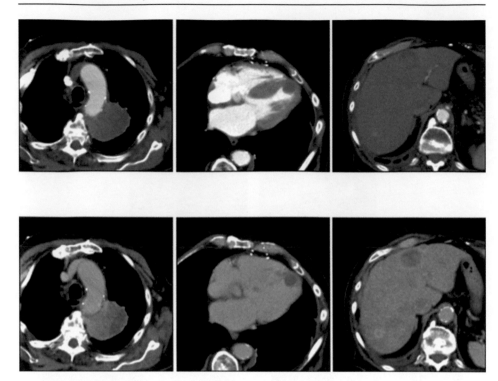

Figure 10.18 Intramural hematoma, differential diagnosis (3). This figure shows images of a patient, who presented with chest pain. The CT shows changes in the area of the aortic arch with an appearance reminding of blood products. The upper panels show images from the arterial phase and the lower panels show delayed venous phase. Careful review in particular of the delayed phase images demonstrates that the lesions are separated from the aortic wall, more consistent with a lung tumour, developing adjacent to the aorta. Supporting a diagnosis of a malignant process, there was evidence of a left ventricular thrombus, and evidence of likely metastatic lesions of the liver (right panels).

whether the presenting pain is from compression of surrounding tissue, particularly of the vertebral bodies, or from leakage (**Figures 10.20** and **10.21**).

10.1.1.4 Differential diagnosis ('triple rule out')

CT scans performed for the assessment of the aorta in patient with suspected AAS allow assessment for other conditions considered in the differential diagnosis, including acute pulmonary embolism or acute coronary syndromes. It has been suggested that CT protocols for patients presenting with acute chest pain could be modified to allow simultaneous assessment of these entities ('triple rule out').[144] However, most experienced centres use a clinically directed diagnostic approach, rather than these non-specific protocols not widely used.[145]

10.1.1.5 Therapeutic implications

Patients with aortic dissection and documented involvement of the ascending aorta are typically evaluated for emergent surgery.[137] However, in certain patient populations, successful initial medical management of Class II IMH of the ascending aorta has been described, but remains controversial.[146–149] The identification of acute complications, in

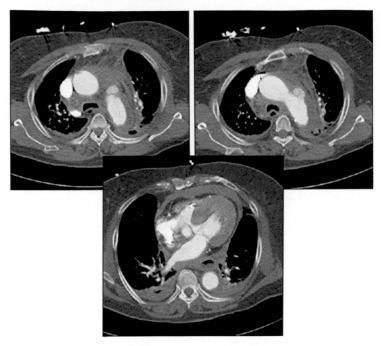

Figure 10.19 Ruptured PAU. These images show a ruptured penetrating atherosclerotic ulceration (PAU) at the distal arch. There are blood products surrounding the aorta and a moderate pericardial effusion.

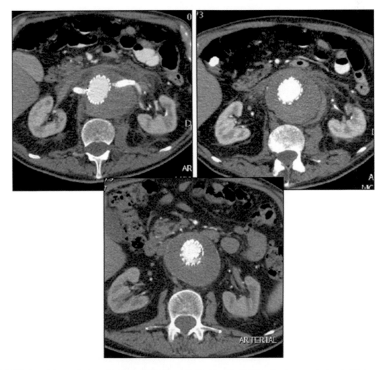

Figure 10.20 Leaking abdominal aneurysm. Patient with AAA prior to renal stent. There are subtle, blood products surrounding the AAA.

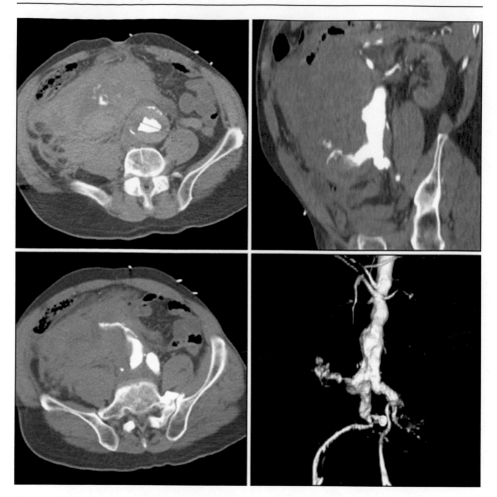

Figure 10.21 Ruptured abdominal aneurysm, active contrast extravasation. Images of a patient presenting to the ED with abdominal pain and hypotension. An emergently performed CT scan demonstrated an abdominal aortic aneurysm with evidence of rupture with active contrast extravasation and large amount of retroperitoneal blood products. The patient was immediately prepared for emergent surgical repair.

particular hemopericardium and mediastinal hematoma, is critical in the management of these patients (**Figures 10.22–10.24**). For patients without involvement of the ascending aorta, initial treatment is typically conservative, with aggressive blood pressure control.[137] However, distal complications including visceral branch vessel compression/ischemia, aortic rupture, intractable pain, and uncontrollable hypertension can require immediate surgical or endovascular treatment (**Figure 10.25**).

10.1.2 Aortic Aneurysmal Disease

CT is routinely performed for the identification and characterization of thoracic and abdominal aortic aneurysmal disease. CT protocols with 1–3 mm slice reconstruction allow precise assessment of the aorta, arch and visceral branch vessels, as well as iliac arteries. CTA shows

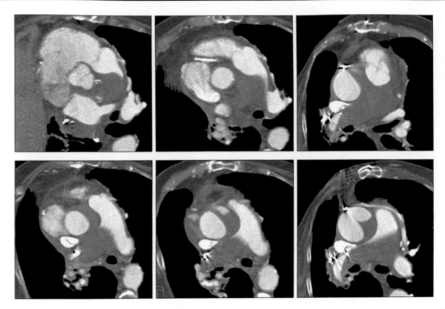

Figure 10.22 Type A aortic dissection with evidence of mediastinal blood products. The images in this figure show an acute type A aortic dissection beginning at the sinotubular junction and extending into the arch. The false channel is partially thrombosed. There is evidence of leakage/rupture with mediastinal blood products, which compresses the right pulmonary artery.

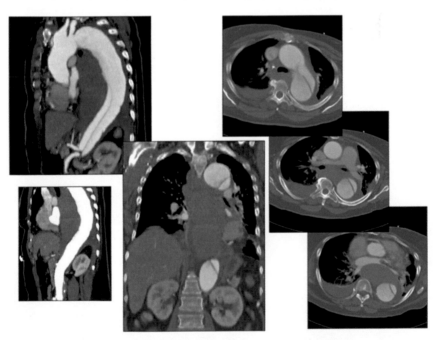

Figure 10.23 Type B aortic dissection with evidence of rupture. This figure shows images of a patient with a type B aortic dissection beginning just beyond the origin of the left subclavian artery. There are luminal irregularities in the aortic isthmus, which may represent the site of tear. The mediastinum is notable for large amount of blood products surrounding the descending thoracic aorta extending to the level of the diaphragm. This is associated with partial compression of the left atrium and pulmonary veins. There are bilateral pleural effusions with increased density consistent with complex and haemorrhagic effusions.

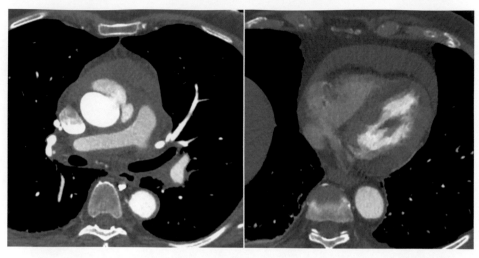

Figure 10.24 Rupture. This figure shows images of a patient with a focal type A dissection limited to the ascending segment. There is a large, haemorrhagic pericardial effusion.

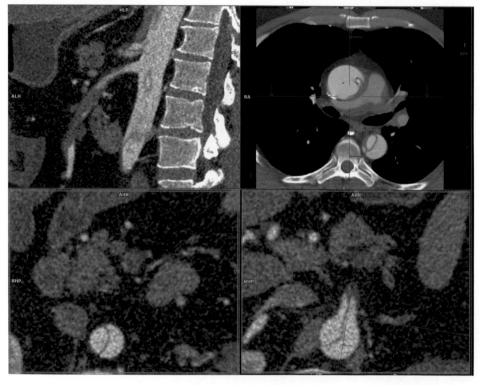

Figure 10.25 Compressed true lumen. This figure shows images of a patient with type A aortic dissection. There is compression of the true lumen in the ascending segment (right upper panel) and thrombosis/occlusion of the SMA (left upper panel).

luminal dimensions and the vessel wall. In aortic aneurysm, luminal dimensions, intraluminal thrombus, and calcification of the aneurysm sac can be assessed. Dimensions of the aneurysm are described by measuring the outer dimensions of the aneurysm sac, which has prognostic and therapeutic implication.

Reconstruction of images perpendicular to the vessel axis for each segment of the aorta allows precise assessment and measurement of aneurysms, e.g. of the sinuses of Valsalva (sinus of Valsalva aneurysm, **Figures 10.26–10.28**), ectasia of the aortic root and ascending aorta (**Figures 10.29** and **10.30**), aneurysms of the descending thoracic aorta (**Figure 10.31**), and aneurysms of the abdominal aorta.

Post-traumatic aneurysms are typically seen in the proximal descending aortic segment. The initial features are those of a focal dissection/transection (**Figure 10.9**). In later stages, there is often focal aneurysmal dilatation with wall calcification (**Figure 10.32**).

An occasional finding with aneurysms typically of the abdominal aorta is a rim of soft tissue (suspected inflammatory tissue). These aneurysms are described as inflammatory aneurysms (**Figure 10.33**).[150] There is an overlap with retroperitoneal fibrosis.

Connective tissue disease including Marfan syndrome is associated with aortic aneurysms and dissection, and skeletal abnormalities (**Figures 10.34** and **10.35**). While CT is typically preferred in particular for diagnosis in symptomatic patient and for treatment planning, MRI of the aorta is the strong alternative modality in particular for younger patients during follow-up, because of its lack of radiation exposure. In most cases, MRA of the aorta can be performed without gadolinium contrast administration.

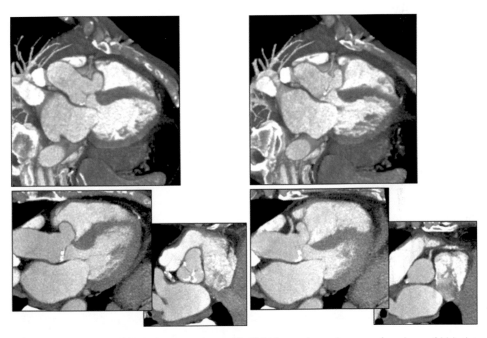

Figure 10.26 Sinus of Valsalva aneurysm (1). This figure shows images of a sinus of Valsalva aneurysm. There is a 1.4 × 2.4 × 1.9 cm saccular outpouching of the right coronary sinus limited to its lower portion immediately above the aortic valve. The RCA arises from the more superior portion of the otherwise normal appearing right coronary sinus of Valsalva.

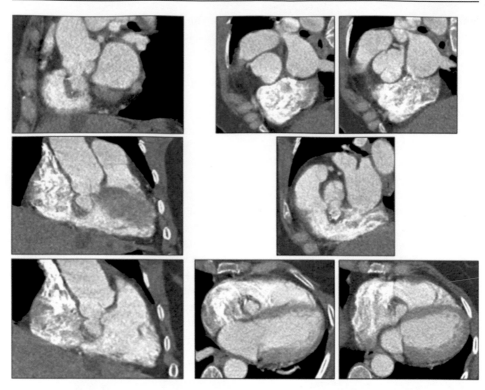

Figure 10.27 Sinus of Valsalva aneurysm (2). Another example of a sinus of Valsalva aneurysm is shown in this figure. It originates from the non-coronary cusp and measures 2.5 × 2.1 cm. It is in close relation to the atria aspect of the sepal leaflet of the tricuspid valve. The aneurysm is partially thrombosed but well perfused in the central portion. No communication is evident.

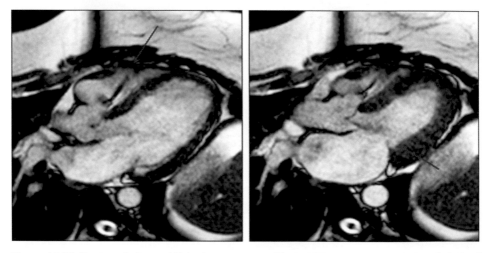

Figure 10.28 Ruptured sinus of Valsalva aneurysm. These MRI images show a ruptured sinus of Valsalva aneurysm, with a jet extending into the RV.

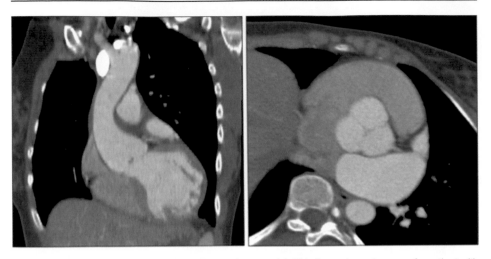

Figure 10.29 Dilated aortic root (annulo-aortic ectasia). This figure shows images of a patient with Marfan syndrome. The aortic valve is trileaflet. There is a dilated aortic root with effacement of sinotubular junction. Beyond the dilated root, the aorta has normal dimensions. The pattern of dilatation is consistent with annulo-aortic ectasia.

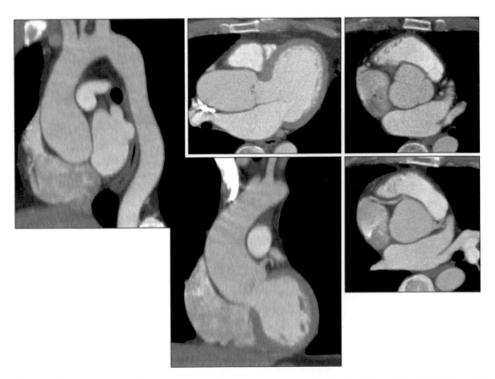

Figure 10.30 Annulo-aortic ectasia. Another example of annulo-aortic ectasia with prominence of aortic root and proximal ascending aorta (maximum diameter 5.2 cm) is shown. There is associated effacement of the sinotubular junction.

143

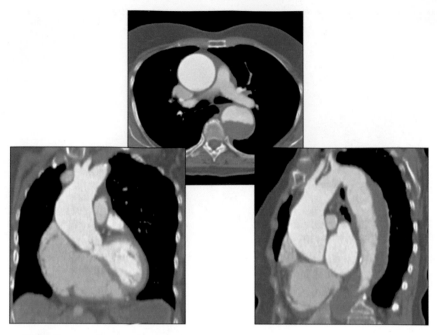

Figure 10.31 Descending aortic aneurysm. This figure shows images of an aortic aneurysm of the descending thoracic aorta with moderate-to-severe amount of adherent wall thrombus. There is also dilatation of the ascending aorta.

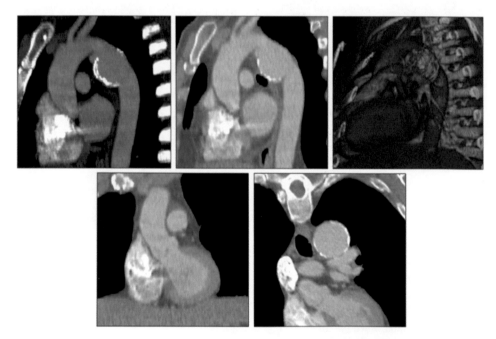

Figure 10.32 Post-traumatic aneurysm. This figure shows images of a patient with a remote history of a motor vehicle accident. There is a focal aneurysm in the area of the isthmus and proximal descending thoracic aorta with eccentric expansion and calcification of its anterolateral surface. Maximum diameter is 4.8 cm. Proximal and distal to the aneurysm, the aorta has normal dimensions and minimal atherosclerotic changes.

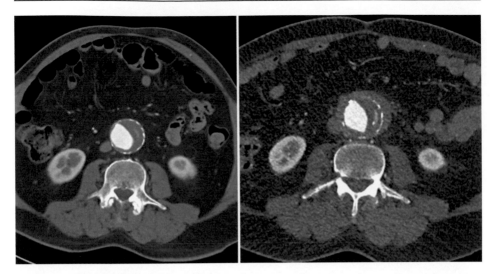

Figure 10.33 Inflammatory aneurysm. This figure shows findings consistent with an inflammatory aneurysm (right panel). Surrounding the calcified outer wall of the aneurysm sac is a rim of soft tissue changes, most consistent with inflammatory changes. The left panel shows the aneurysm from a prior CT scan, which had been obtained 3 years earlier.

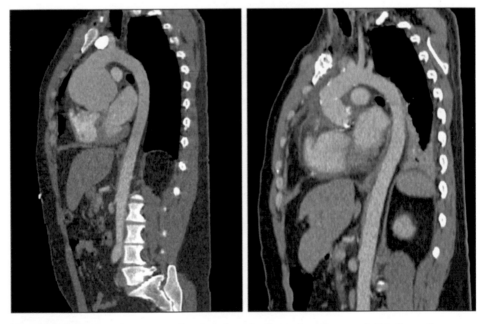

Figure 10.34 Pre- and postoperative imaging: Aortic root replacement. This figure shows pre- and postoperative images of a aneurysmally dilated ascending aorta. There is massive dilatation of the aortic root and proximal ascending aorta with a maximum diameter of 8 cm (left panel). The postoperative CT (right panel) demonstrates replacement of the aortic valve, and sequential grafts covering the aortic root, ascending aorta, and parts of the aortic arch.

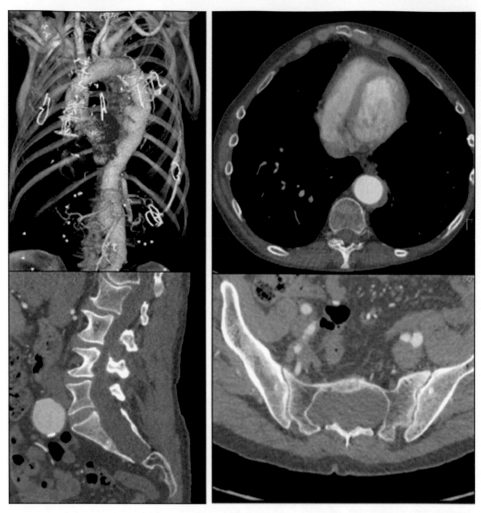

Figure 10.35 Extracardiac findings with Marfan syndrome. This patient with a history of Marfan syndrome had undergone prior aortic surgery. The surgical grafts are shown in the left upper panel in a volume-rendered image (VRI). The right upper panel demonstrates pectus deformity of the chest. The left and right lower panels show dural ectasia of the sacrum.

10.1.3 Endovascular Stent Graft

CT imaging of the aorta is an integral part of endovascular stent graft therapy of aortic aneurysms.[151–154] CT is critical for procedural planning, with detailed 3-D reconstructions used for precise quantitative assessment for custom-made stent grafts (**Figures 10.36–10.41**). It is also an integral part of post-procedural surveillance.

10.1.4 Aortic Surgery

Pre- and postoperative CT scans are useful for surgical planning and in the assessment of surgical results (**Figures 10.42–10.44**) and early and late complications. In the early

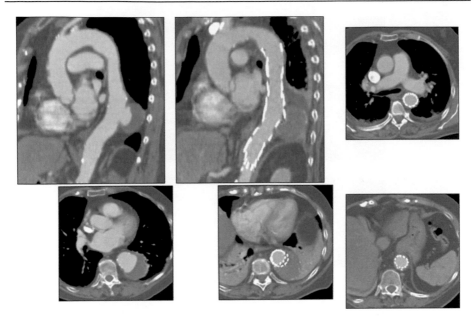

Figure 10.36 Endovascular stent graft. This figure shows images of a patient with a focal pseudoaneurysm/PAU of the descending thoracic aorta (left upper and lower panels). The aorta at the level of the pseudoaneurysm measures 6.9 × 5.0 cm. The patient was treated with an endovascular stent graft (middle and right panels). The endovascular stent graft series extends from the proximal descending thoracic aorta to the level just above the celiac artery. The stent successfully excludes the aneurysm sac of the retrocardiac descending thoracic aorta. There is no endoleak.

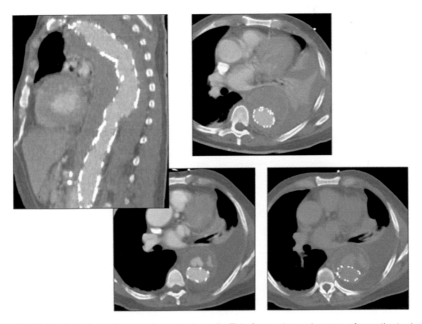

Figure 10.37 Endoleak endovascular stent graft. This figure shows images of a patient who was treated with a repeat endovascular stent procedure because of endoleak. The lower images show the areas of endoleak after the initial procedure (left lower: arterial phase; right lower: venous phase). After repeat stenting no leak is seen in the same area (upper panels).

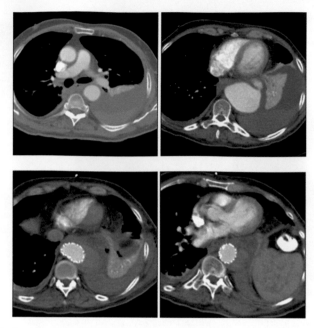

Figure 10.38 Endovascular stent graft, ruptured aneurysm. These images show a ruptured aneurysm at the level of the retrocardiac descending thoracic aorta (left upper panels). There is contrast extravasation in the anterior aspect of the aneurysm and evidence of a haemmorhagic left pleural effusion. The patient was treated emergently with a thoracoabdominal endovascular stent graft (left lower panels and right panel).

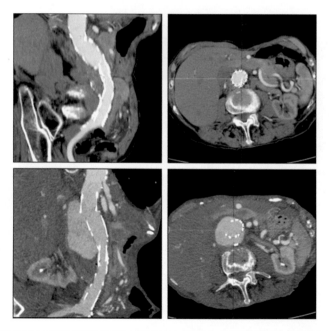

Figure 10.39 Endovascular stent graft, stent separation, endoleak (1). Images of a patient with prior endovascular stent grafting of the abdominal aorta. The upper images show baseline images, the lower images were obtained at the time of presentation with abdominal pain. There is evidence of separation of stent components with an associated large endoleak.

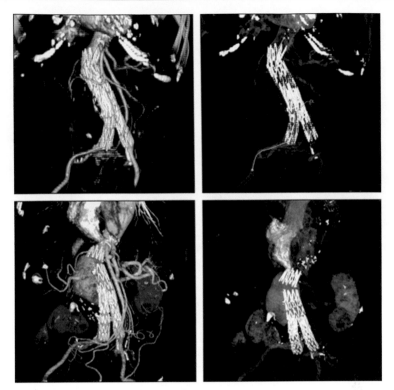

Figure 10.40 Endovascular stent graft, stent separation, endoleak (2). This figure shows volume-rendered images (VRIs) baseline (upper panels) and follow-up (lower panels), demonstrating the stent component separation.

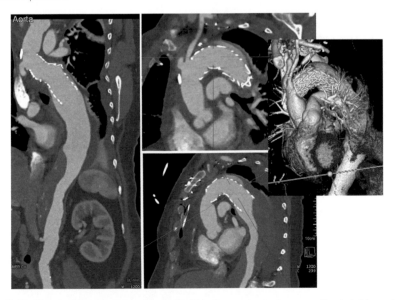

Figure 10.41 'Frozen elephant-trunk' graft. This figure shows images after hybrid surgical and endovascular repair of the ascending aorta and arch. There is a supra-coronary surgical graft of the ascending aorta, which is continuous with an endovascular stent graft of the distal arch and proximal descending aorta.

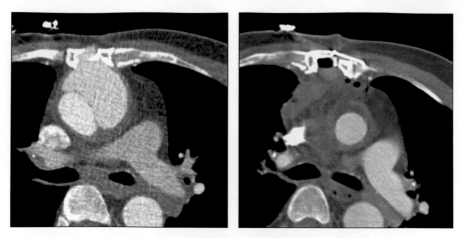

Figure 10.42 Preoperative assessment of sternal anatomy. Images of a patient with a history of type A aortic dissection, which was in the past repaired with a short supra-coronary graft of the ascending aorta. The patient developed a pseudoaneurysm at the level of the distal anastomosis site. The left panel shows preoperative images of the level of the mid-ascending aorta, with the pseudoaneurysm anterior to the surgical graft. The anterior aspect of the pseudoaneurysm lies immediately against the posterior wall of the sternum and appears to extend into the gap between the sternal halves (poststernotomy with sternal malunion). This information was critical in planning the access approach for the planned redo median sternotomy and aortic cannulation (a femoral cannulation approach was chosen). The right panel shows the same level after redo open-heart surgery. A new graft of the ascending aorta is surrounded by postoperative blood products and small amounts of air.

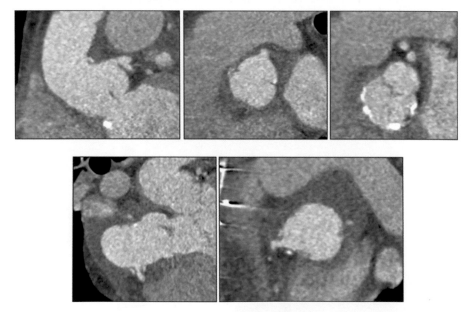

Figure 10.43 Aortic root repair. This figure shows images of a patient with aortic root repair. Only the non- and right-coronary sinus of Valsalva was replaced with a surgical graft. The native left sinus of Valsalva was maintained. Therefore, only the right coronary artery was re-implanted. The native aortic valve was re-suspended in a modified David procedure. The origin of the native left main coronary artery of the left sinus of Valsalva is shown in the upper panels. The upper right panel shows high-density surgical material adjacent to the replaced non- and right-sinus of Valsalva. The lower panels show the re-implanted right coronary artery, with surgical material at the coronary button.

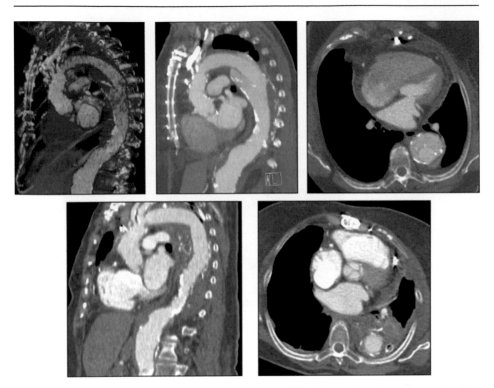

Figure 10.44 Surgical graft, 'elephant-trunk procedure'. The 'elephant-trunk procedure' describes a two-stage surgical technique for patients with extensive aneurysmal disease of the thoracic aorta. In the first stage (via median sternotomy), the ascending aorta and/or aortic root are replaced with a surgical graft. An additional surgical graft is anastomosed at the isthmus and left hanging freely in the dilated descending aorta. In the second stage of the procedure, the free distal end of the graft is anastomosed to the descending aorta (via a left thoracotomy), excluding the dilated descending aorta. This figure shows postoperative images of a patient after the first (upper panels) and the second (lower panels) stages of an 'elephant-trunk procedure.' The upper images show surgical grafts of most of the ascending aorta and continuation of the graft, freely hanging into the proximal descending aorta. There are metallic markers at the distal end of the graft, which are also seen in the cross-sectional image (right upper panel). The graft inside the dilated proximal descending thoracic aorta can be confused with a dissection, if the surgical history is not known. In the second stage of the 'elephant-trunk procedure,' the free end of the graft was connected to the mid-descending aorta, with excision of the dilated proximal descending aorta. (Compare to **Figure 10.41** of a 'Frozen elephant-trunk' graft.)

postoperative phase, complications at the repair site or in the operative field, including mediastinal hematoma or infection (**Figures 10.45–10.47**), pericardial or pleural effusion, and pneumothorax, can be identified. Late complications include prosthetic valve graft infections, postoperative pseudoaneurysms, and fistulas after surgery (**Figures 10.48–10.51**).

10.1.5 Non-Aortic Preoperative Imaging

An important application of CT is perioperative imaging of the aorta in patients undergoing cardiothoracic surgery.[155,156] In patients undergoing open-heart surgery,

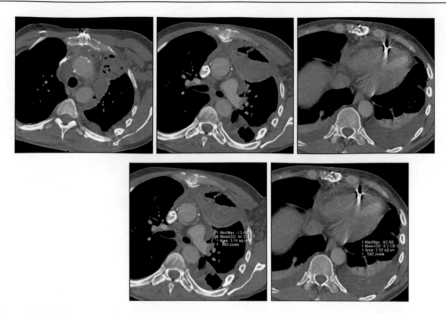

Figure 10.45 Postoperative empyema. This figure shows images of a patient with a remote history of aortic valve replacement and recent bacterial endocarditis. Ten days before the CT scan, the patient underwent replacement of the aortic valve and ascending thoracic aorta using a composite graft. The patient remained febrile and demonstrated and elevated white blood count. The CT scan shows evidence of aortic valve replacement and replacement of the ascending thoracic aorta with a composite graft. The graft is surrounded by the expected postoperative blood products. There is a small-size right-sided and a moderate-size left-sided pleural effusion with adjacent atelectasis. There is a large air/fluid collection measuring 13 × 7 cm in the left upper pleural space, most consistent with an abscess. There are small mediastinal lymph nodes and prominent axillary lymph nodes.

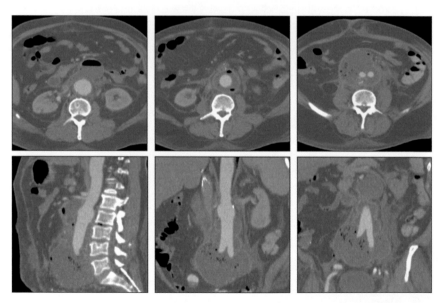

Figure 10.46 Infected abdominal surgical graft. This figure shows images of patient several days after placement of an infrarenal aorto-bifemoral graft. There is a large perigraft fluid collection consistent with graft infection. The more superior fluid collection with a prominent air fluid level suggests the possibility of an aorto-enteric fistula as the source of the infection.

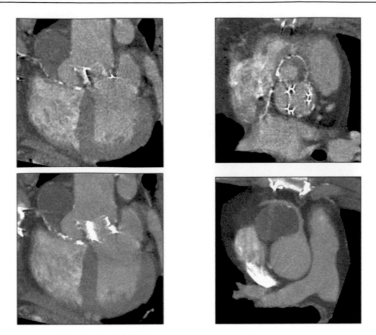

Figure 10.47 Postoperative pseudoaneurysm. This figure shows images of a patient with remote aortic valve replacement for endocarditis and pericardial patch repair of a subcoronary abscess cavity. The patch had partially dehisced generating a supra-annular/subcoronary pseudoaneurysm. The CT demonstrates a partially thrombosed pseudoaneurysm of the aortic root at right sinus of Valsalva (arrow). The right coronary artery (RCA) is draped over the pseudoaneurysm (right lower panel).

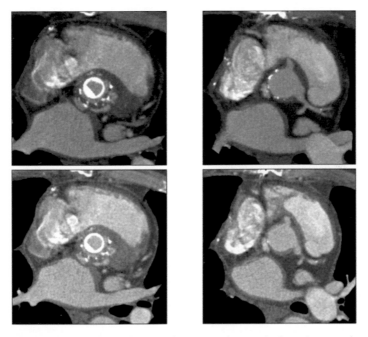

Figure 10.48 Root abscess. A smaller pseudoaneurysm is seen in these images of a patient that underwent placement of a composite surgical graft of the root and ascending aorta with aortic valve replacement (mechanical valve). Small contrast-filled cavities are seen (right lower panel).

153

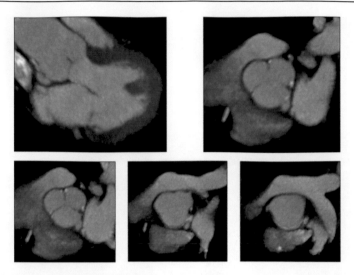

Figure 10.49 Postoperative pseudoaneurysm. This figure shows images of a patient with remote placement of a supra-coronary graft of the aorta for type A aortic dissection repair. There is a prominent native aortic root measuring 4.2 cm and a supra-coronary graft of the ascending aorta. There is a small saccular outpouching at the proximal anastomosis adjacent to the non-coronary sinus of Valsalva consistent with a pseudoaneurysm (upper panels). Suture material at the proximal anastomosis of the supra-coronary graft of the ascending aorta is demonstrated (right lower panel).

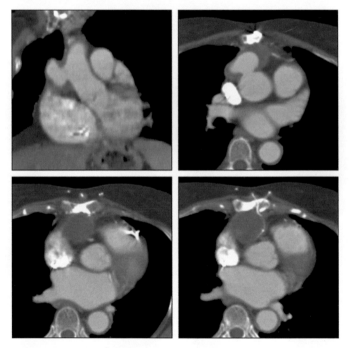

Figure 10.50 Mycotic pseudoaneurysm of the ascending aorta. This figure shows images of a patient who developed a mycotic pseudoaneurysm after mitral valve repair. Residuals of retained epicardial pacer wires are seen in the subcutaneous tissue of the anterior chest wall (right lower panel). There is a small amount of subcutaneous fluid surrounding the wire. There is a presumably mycotic pseudoaneurysm arising from the mid-ascending aorta, in a retrosternal location. The saccular outpouching measures 3.6 × 4.7 × 4.7 cm and is partially thrombus filled (upper panels).

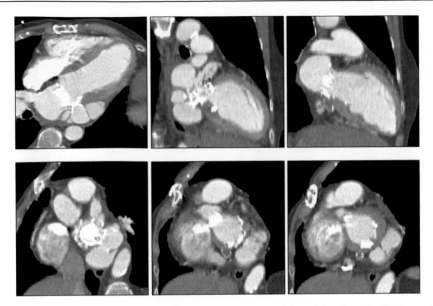

Figure 10.51 Postoperative pseudoaneurysm of left ventricle originating at mitral annulus.
This figure shows images of a patient with a remote history of aortic and mitral valve replacement, with mechanical valves. Originating from the inferolateral and lateral aspect of the mitral annulus is a contrast-filled space measuring 6.5 × 4.8 cm. It extends along the lateral wall of the left atrium and basal segments of the left ventricle. Its borders are partially calcified. It communicates at the level of the mitral valve prosthesis with left ventricle. In addition, there is a small outpouching originating from the inferior aspect of the mitral annulus, which is thrombosed and has calcification of the wall. It measures 1.0 × 1.9 cm.

the local extent of calcified atherosclerotic plaque of the ascending aorta determines the cannulation site during cardiopulmonary bypass. If extensive plaque and calcification preclude cannulation of the ascending aorta, a temporarily placed bypass conduit to the axillary or subclavian artery is a frequently used alternative. To assess for calcification, a non–contrast-enhanced CT scan is sufficient, but does not allow to assess non-calcified atherosclerotic changes. Contrast-enhanced scans show the amount of calcified and non-calcified atherosclerotic plaque, which is related to postoperative stroke incidence and outcome.[157,158]

10.1.6 Other Conditions

Occasionally, CT demonstrates changes consistent with thrombus protruding into the aortic lumen. Thrombus may develop on the luminal surface of intimal changes (**Figure 10.52**).

Morphologic changes associated with aortitis can be assessed with CT. Typical findings in the acute setting are wall thickening (**Figure 10.53**) and branch vessel stenosis. In chronic stages, branch vessel stenosis and extensive calcification are seen. The role of positron emission tomography (PET)/CT in the assessment of disease activity is incompletely understood (**Figure 10.54**). Isolated aortitis describes a clinical scenario where histologic evidence of aortitis is identified in surgical samples after aortic surgery,

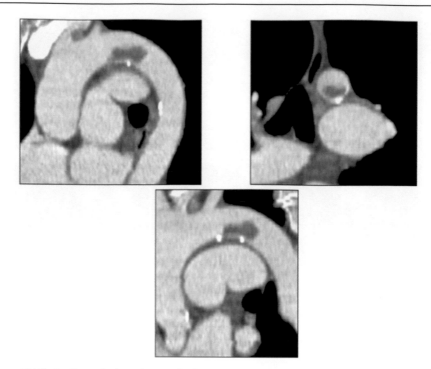

Figure 10.52 Aortic arch thrombus and atheroma. This figure shows a protruding soft tissue in the aortic arch, consistent with thrombus. There is underlying calcified atherosclerotic plaque.

but no clinical symptoms of vasculitis are present. In these patients, diffuse aortic dilatation has been described.[159,160]

An incidental finding of an intra-aortic balloon pump in the aorta is shown in **Figure 10.55**. Aortic coarctation is further described in Chapter 13 (Section 13.6, 'Aortic Disease') on congenital disease (Chapter 11).

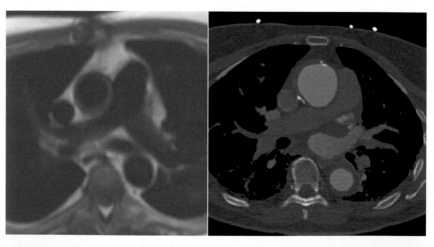

Figure 10.53 Aortitis. This figure shows MRI (left panel) and ST (right panel) of patient with aortitis. In both images, thickening of the ascending aorta is identified. The patient had known history of vasculitis and presented with elevated serum inflammatory markers.

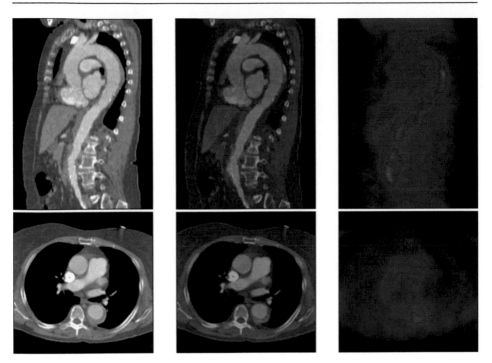

Figure 10.54 Aortitis, positron emission tomography (PET)/CT. This figure shows MDCT and PET images of a patient with aortitis. The CT (left panels) demonstrates smooth wall thickening of the aorta compatible with aortitis. There is prominent wall thickening in the mid-lower descending thoracic aorta with a maximum thickness of 1.2 cm. There is also prominent wall thickening of the aorta at the renal artery level, which is indistinguishable from a large amount of para-aortic soft tissue. The metabolic PET images (right panels) demonstrate regions of moderately intense fluorodeoxyglucose (FDG) uptake associated with the descending thoracic aorta and segments of the abdominal aorta. These findings are consistent with hypermetabolic inflammatory changes involving the aorta. Fusion images (middle panels) combine the anatomic and functional information.

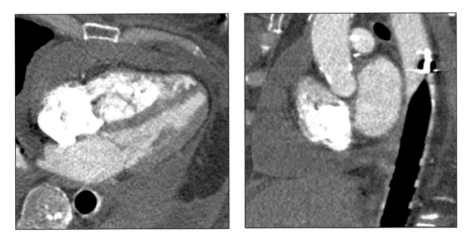

Figure 10.55 Intra-aortic balloon pump. This figure shows images of a patient with a pericardial effusion. In the descending aorta, an intra-aortic balloon pump is seen. In the late diastolic images, the inflated balloon is seen in cross-sectional (left panel) and longitudinal (right panel) images. Additional image reconstruction in systole (during balloon deflation) allows better visualization of the aortic wall.

Peripheral Artery Disease

11.1 Peripheral Artery Disease

Because of their relatively large size, lack of motion, and straight course, assessment of peripheral arteries, including the identification and quantification of luminal stenosis, can be performed with CT angiography (CTA) (**Figure 11.1**). Vessel wall calcification remains a major limitation in particular in smaller vessels. MDCT protocols typically use a spiral examination mode with thin, overlapping images and rapid contrast bolus injection. CTA has developed into an alternative imaging modality in several vascular regions. The experience in lower extremity peripheral artery disease (PAD) imaging is described next. The assessment of subclavian artery access in the context of TAVR is discussed in Chapter 7. In neuroradiology, modern systems allow simultaneous imaging of the carotid arteries, intracranial vessel, brain morphology, and brain perfusion. CTA is also increasingly being used for the assessment of renal artery disease, carotid disease, and atherosclerotic disease of the lower-extremity arteries, often as a 'road-map' for subsequent angioplasty. Disadvantages of CT in comparison with ultrasound and MRI are the associated radiation exposure and the lack of flow information.

11.1.1 Lower Extremity CTA

CTA of the entire lower extremity arterial system, which includes supra-inguinal inflow vessels and infra-inguinal runoff, has only become possible with the introduction of multidetector-row CT and has largely replaced diagnostic intra-arterial angiography. The most important indication for lower extremity CTA is treatment planning in patients with PAD.[161,162] Other indications include acute ischemia, trauma, and anatomic imaging, such as before free-flap harvesting, or in athletes suspected of functional or anatomic popliteal entrapment syndrome, or iliac endofibrosis. The role of lower extremity CTA in the setting of PAD is not necessarily to establish the diagnosis, which is typically based on symptoms, clinical exam, and noninvasive testing such as ankle-brachial index. The strength of lower extremity CTA is to map the disease process within this large territory, which is critical for treatment planning.

The anatomic coverage for a lower extremity CT angiogram typically extends from T12 (if suprarenal aorta is to be included) down to the toes, with a relatively small field-of-view (SOV), in order to maintain adequate in-plane resolution. Through-plane resolution (in the z-axis) is typically 0.7–1.25 mm. While lower extremity CTA, data acquisition is relatively straightforward with state-of-the-art equipment, synchronization with contrast medium delivery requires particular attention to the fact that bolus propagation in a diseased lower

DOI: 10.1201/9781003153641-13

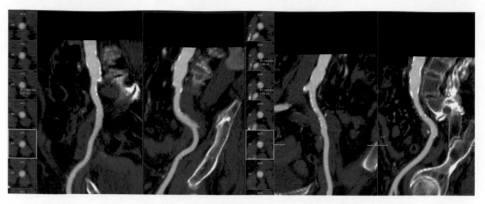

Figure 11.1 Iliac arteries. This figure shows centreline reconstructions of the left and right iliac arteries.

extremity arterial tree may be substantially delayed. This may require use of a relatively long scan time and preparing for an optional second pass from above the knees down through the toes.[163]

A challenging component of lower extremity CTA is visualization and post-processing of the typically 1,000–2,000 axial CT images. Analysis is often limited by significant vessel wall calcifications or stents in place. Analysis techniques include curved planar reformations (CPR), either through each arterial branch separately, or as so-called multi-path CPR (**Figures 11.2** and **11.3**).[164] Processing of lower extremity CTA may be time consuming, and large programs might benefit from dedicated technologists or a 3-D laboratory to generate standardized images of the lower extremity arterial tree.

Lower extremity CTA is an accurate imaging modality in patients with intermittent claudication, with a sensitivity of 95% (95% CI, 92–97%), a specificity of 96% (95% CI, 93–97%) for detecting more than 50% stenosis or occlusions reported in a prior meta-analysis.[165] CTA is more accurate than Doppler ultrasound, and performs equal or better than MRA.[166] The accuracy of lower extremity CTA decreases in below-knee vessels, with the main limiting factor being the presence of arterial calcifications. However, CTA provides accurate recommendations for the management of patients with critical limb ischemia as well.[167]

Dual-energy CT technology allows differentiation of iodine from calcium and is used in the context of PAD.[168]

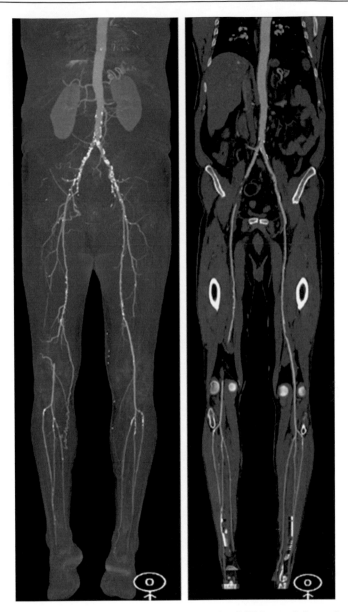

Figure 11.2 Lower leg CTA (1). Maximum intensity projection (MIP) image (left panel) and multi-path curved planar reformation (right panel) of a lower extremity CTA obtained in a 55-year-old man with a 10-year history of claudication and an ankle-brachial index of 0.5 on the right, and 0.8 on the left. Moderate atherosclerotic calcification in the MIP image (left) preclude assessment of suprainguinal vessels. Multi-path curved planar reformation (right) clearly shows a 6 cm occlusion of the right external iliac artery. Collateral vessels (via an obturator artery) are shown in the MIP image (left). Both, the MIP image (left) and the mpCPR show a well collateralized 9 cm distal superficial femoral artery occlusion. On the left, there are approximately 50% focal stenosis at the external iliac arteries, and more than 50% stenosis of the superficial femoral artery at the level of the adductor hiatus. Crural arteries are patent.

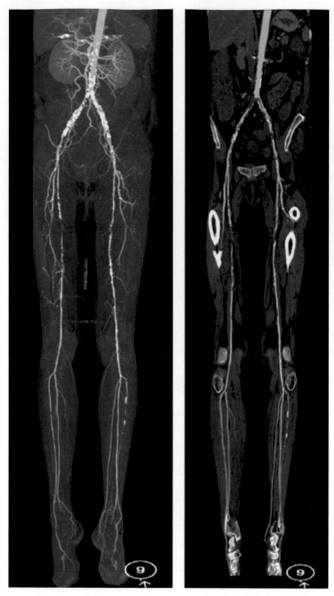

Figure 11.3 Lower leg CTA (2). Maximum intensity projection (MIP) image (left) and multi-path curved planar reformation (mpCPR) of a lower extremity CT angiogram obtained in a 69-year-old woman with right lower extremity ischemia and gangrenous toes. Extensive atherosclerotic calcification of the aorto-iliac vasculature in the MIP (left) image obscure a short complete occlusion of the right common iliac artery, and extensive stenosis of the bilateral suprainguinal system, as shown in the mpCPR (right). The right superficial femoral artery is diffusely diseased and occluded, and reconstitutes in the distal thigh. The anterior tibial artery below the knee is moderately diseased and patent. Congenitally absent posterior tibial artery with compensatory enlargement of a patent, proximally diseased peroneal artery. Multiple stenoses are also seen in the left superficial femoral artery. The left anterior tibial artery is completely occluded.

12

Cardiac Masses

Cardiac masses are typically initially imaged with echocardiography, MRI, and PET/SPECT. However, CT provides valuable anatomic information is selected patients. It is e.g. superior in defining the relationship of lung masses to the pericardium and heart,[169] and may allow to define blood supply of cardiac masses. If dedicated CT imaging is planned, the protocol should be modified for the specific clinical question. If a mass with suspected mobility is evaluated, retrospective gated acquisition modes, optimally on scanners with high temporal resolution, should be used to limit motion artefact (**Figures 12.1** and **12.2**). The anatomic criteria seldom allow a definitive 'histologic' diagnosis, but rather to differentiate between likely benign versus malignant lesions, with implications for further management.

Cardiac masses are described with regard to size, location, and spatial relationship to adjacent structures. It is important to evaluate the border of the mass (capsulated, well-defined, irregular, infiltrative), the density (HU) of the mass, its homogeneity, and contrast enhancement after contrast administration. A dedicated protocol similar to a coronary acquisition may also define details of blood supply (**Figures 12.4**, **12.13**, and **12.16**). Similar to MRI, which allows superior tissue characterization, classification of masses according to these criteria allows to associate certain patterns with corresponding masses.[170–172] As described above, an important clinical question is the differentiation between likely benign and malignant processes. Imaging can provide important clues, but the definitive diagnosis requires surgical sampling and pathology. From the wide variety of primary benign and malignant cardiac tumours and cardiac metastasis, the following examples of benign and malignant tumours demonstrate basic imaging criteria.

Common benign tumours are atrial myxomas. Myxomas often originate from the left atrium or mitral annulus with a stalk, and may demonstrate tumour calcification (**Figures 12.1** and **12.2**). However, as described above, definitive characterization is often not possible with CT imaging alone (**Figures 12.3–12.6**). Benign masses of the left ventricle have similar characteristics, and additional MRI is often utilized for further characterization (**Figures 12.7** and **12.8**).

Signs of malignancy, which can be assessed with CT, include infiltration of adjacent structures and the presence of tumour vessels. Examples are shown in **Figures 12.9–12.18**.

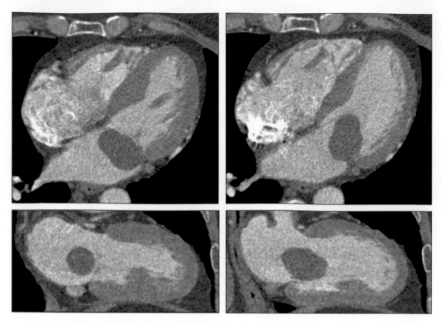

Figure 12.1 Atrial myxoma (1). the images in this figure show an atrial tumour, consistent with a myxoma. The mass appears to be broadly attached in the area of the posterior mitral annulus and measures 2.8 × 2.8 × 3.7 cm. It is non-calcified and homogeneous and shows no evidence of enhancement.

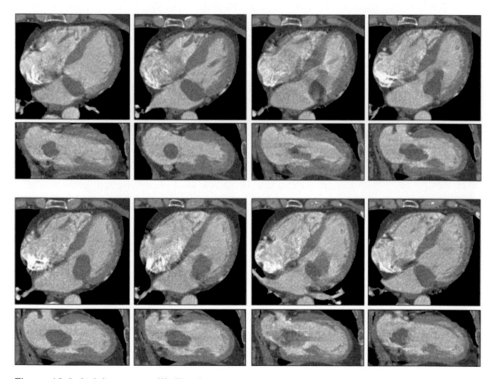

Figure 12.2 Atrial myxoma (2). This figure shows multiple reconstructions of the mass at different phases of the cardiac cycle. The images demonstrate that the mobile tumour passes through the valve plane during diastole.

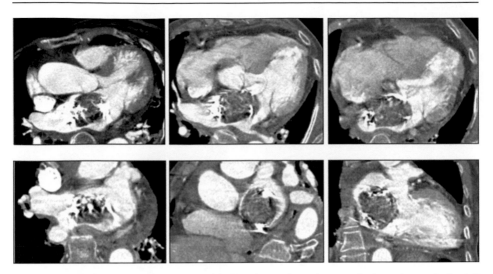

Figure 12.3 Suspected atrial myxoma (1). This figure shows images of a large tumour in the left atrium, attached with a broad base to the intraatrial septum. The tumour is partially calcified. The findings are suggestive of atrial myxoma.

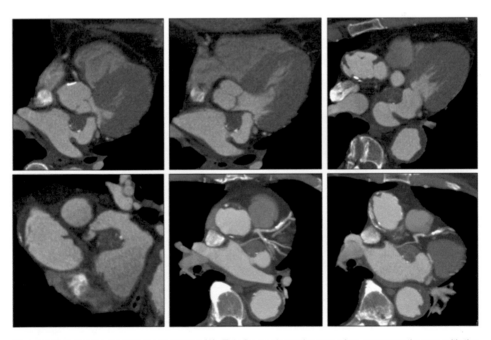

Figure 12.4 Suspected atrial myxoma (2). This figure shows images of a tumour contiguous with the roof of the left atrial body near the origin of the atrial appendage. The tissue is slightly heterogeneous with internal calcification and mildly enhancement, measuring 2.0 × 1.6 × 1.7 cm. Originating from the proximal circumflex artery is an atrial branch, which extends into the region of the mass of the left atrium. Although these findings are most consistent with atrial myxoma with atypical location, definitive characterization is not possible.

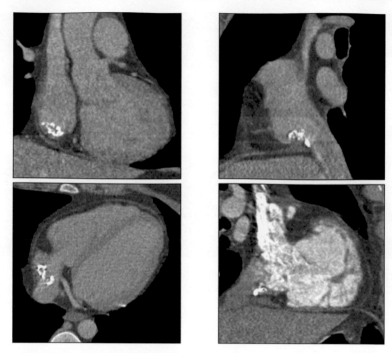

Figure 12.5 Calcified right atrial thrombus. This figure shows images of a patient with a history of Hodgkin disease. Image acquisition was delayed in relation to the contrast injection to avoid contrast streak artefacts in the right atrium. At the inferior wall of the right atrium close to the junction with the inferior vena cava is a small tissue mound, which extends over a distance of 2 cm and has a thickness of 0.8 cm. There is calcification of the tissue. The appearance suggests a benign process, most likely a calcified thrombus, secondary to trauma from a central line.

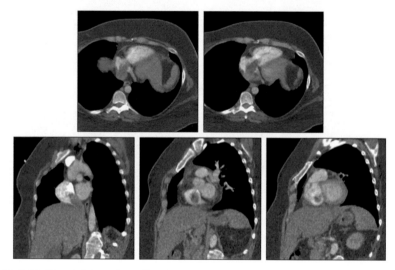

Figure 12.6 Right atrial thrombus. This figure shows images of a low-density mass extending from the inferior vena cava (IVC) near the confluence of the hepatic veins to the level of the tricuspid valve. The mass does not appear to occlude the IVC or the right-sided atrioventricular inflow. Its low attenuation suggests thrombus. The cardiac chambers are otherwise unremarkable. The kidneys are intact and there is no evidence of renal malignancy. The patient underwent excision of the mass. Pathology was consistent with an organizing thrombus.

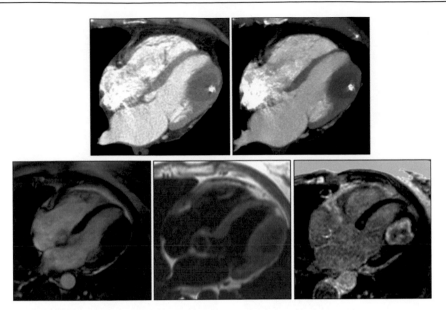

Figure 12.7 Suspected left ventricular fibroma (1). A relatively large mass of the lateral left ventricular wall is shown. The CT (upper panels) shows inhomogeneity and a small calcification. The MRI images (lower panels) are shown in comparison. The images in the right lower panel demonstrate contrast enhancement after gadolinium administration. Based on these findings, a fibroma of the left ventricle was suspected.

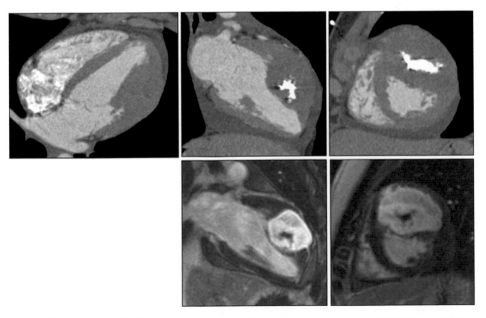

Figure 12.8 Suspected left ventricular fibroma (2). Another example of a suspected left ventricular fibroma is shown in this figure. CT images (upper panels) and MRI images (lower panels) are shown in comparison. Within the anteroapical region of the left ventricle is a mass measuring 4 × 4.7 × 5.8 cm. The lesion is well circumscribed without evidence of surrounding edema or neovascularity. The findings suggest dense fibrotic tissue with focal areas of calcification. The patient subsequently underwent surgery with excision of the mass. Pathology confirmed the diagnosis of a cardiac fibroma.

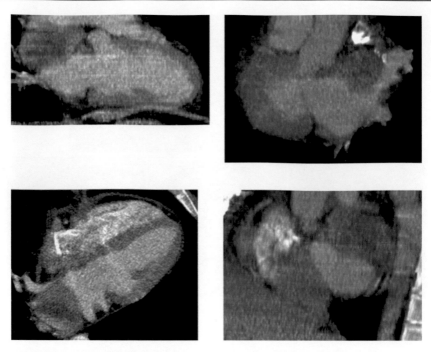

Figure 12.9 **Left atrial paraganglioma (1).** This and the next figure show pre- and postoperative images of a tumour at the roof of the left atrium. The patient underwent surgery and an intraoperative biopsy was consistent with an intrapericardial paraganglioma situated on roof of left atrium. The tumour was subsequently removed.

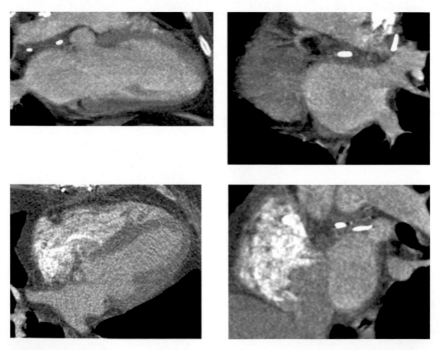

Figure 12.10 **Left atrial paraganglioma (2).** Images at follow-up did not show evidence of residual or recurrent tumour. Surgical clips are seen in the operative field.

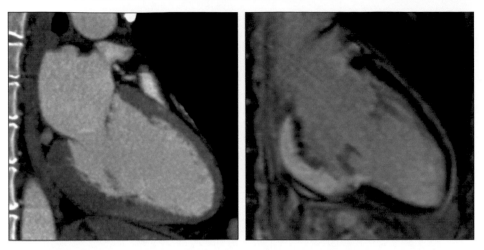

Figure 12.11 Fibrous tumour vs. sarcoidosis (1). This and the next figure show images from a patient presenting with ventricular arrhythmia. The imaging studies demonstrate a fibrous mass of the inferior wall of the left ventricle. Infiltration of the basal inferior wall of the left ventricle is demonstrated with delayed contrast-enhanced MRI imaging (right panel). The same area shows faint hypo-enhancement on the MDCT image.

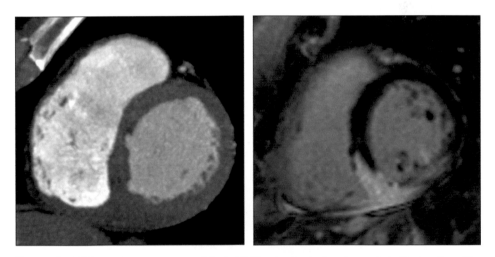

Figure 12.12 Fibrous tumour vs. sarcoidosis (2). The short-axis view demonstrated the location of the tumour of the left ventricle, extending into the right ventricle. Further work-up of the patient demonstrated active sarcoidosis. His clinical symptoms and imaging findings improved during immunosuppressive therapy.

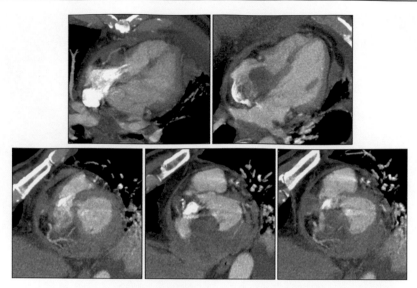

Figure 12.13 Right atrial spindle cell sarcoma. The figure shows images of a tumour of the right atrium. Several small tumour vessels are seen extending into the lesion. The patient underwent surgery with removal of the tumour. Pathology was consistent with a high-grade spindle cell sarcoma.

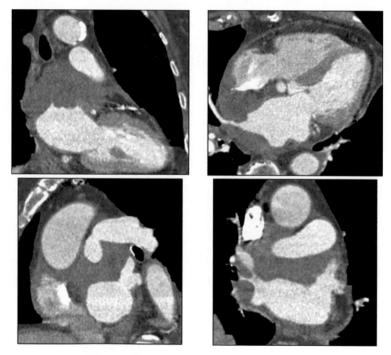

Figure 12.14 Cardiac lymphoma. This figure shows images of a patient with lymphoma. There is a large mediastinal tumour with predominantly intra-pericardial location. It involves the intraatrial septum and the posterior and superior walls of the left and right atria. The tumour encases the pulmonary veins, with partial compression of the right superior vein ostium. In addition, the tumour encases the superior vena cava, left main coronary artery, proximal left anterior descending artery, and proximal left circumflex artery without causing significant compression. Pathology was consistent with a diffuse primary mediastinal diffuse large B-cell lymphoma.

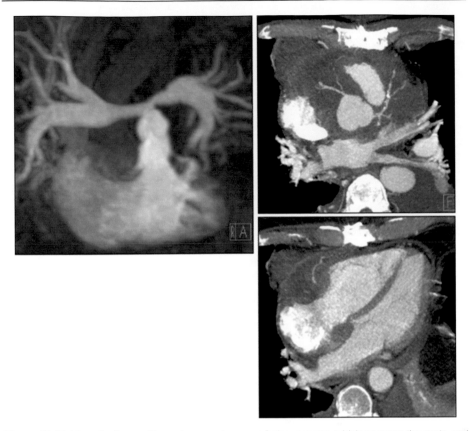

Figure 12.15 Mesothelioma. These images show a soft tissue mass, which encases the aorta and central pulmonary arteries. The narrowing of the central pulmonary arteries is shown in the MRA (left upper panel). There is additional encasement and narrowing of the left superior pulmonary vein. The tumour also involves the right atrial wall and the inflow portion of the right ventricle with suspected myocardial invasion. It extends through the pericardium in the area of the right atrioventricular groove, with complete encasement of the dominant RCA. Pathology was consistent with a malignant spindle cell neoplasm consistent with sarcomatoid mesothelioma.

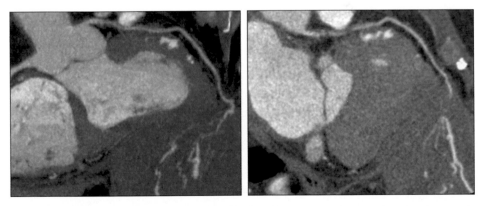

Figure 12.16 Pericardial sarcoma. The identification of tumour vessels, as a sign of malignancy, is often possible secondary to the high-spatial resolution of MDCT. This figure shows images of a large pericardial synovial sarcoma at the inferior aspect of the heart. The CT demonstrated tumour vessels extending from the apical LAD into the tumour.

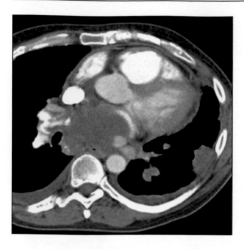
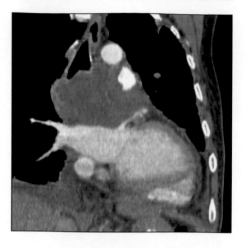

Figure 12.17 Pulmonary artery intimal sarcoma. This figure shows images of a patient with pulmonary artery intimal sarcoma. The initial presentation was shortness of breath, secondary to occlusion of pulmonary artery branches (left panel). The CT scan demonstrates extension into the mediastinum and left atrium, which was confirmed at autopsy.

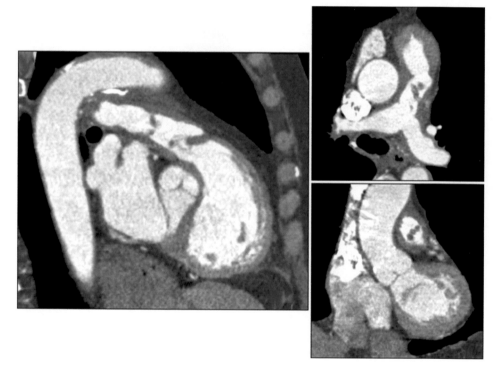

Figure 12.18 Suspected neoplastic involvement of pulmonary artery. This figure shows images from a patient with chest discomfort and worsening shortness of breath. The pulmonary valve demonstrates a nodular appearance. There are mobile nodular lesions of the main pulmonary arteries (arrows). The walls of the pulmonary arteries are markedly thickened confluent with the abnormal increase of tissue of the mediastinum. Additional lung lesions were observed. A malignant process was suspected.

13

Adult Congenital Heart Disease

MDCT is increasingly used in paediatric patients. Because of its short acquisition time, CT can frequently be performed with mild sedation. However, because of the radiation exposure, a particularly careful evaluation of the risks and benefits is necessary in the paediatric patient population.[173,174]

Consistent with the overall focus of the book, this section mainly describes congenital abnormalities, which are seen in adult populations.

13.1 Cardiac Chambers and Myocardium

Atrial septal defects (ASDs) are common congenital heart defects. The different types of defects (ostium secundum defect, ostium primum defect, sinus venosus defect, coronary sinus defect, and patent foramen ovale (PFO) are related to the embryonal development of the intraatrial septum. Unrepaired defects are occasionally identified in asymptomatic or symptomatic adults. Symptoms can include right heart failure or neurologic symptoms secondary to paradoxical embolization. Because the central intraatrial septum is a very thin structure, anatomic assessment with noninvasive imaging modalities is limited. Identification of these defects typically relies on the assessment of flow by echocardiography and MRI. Anatomic assessment with CT can define the relationship of the defect to other anatomic structures, such as the coronary sinus or the sinus venosus (**Figure 13.1**). Surgical or percutaneous closure of ASD is considered, depending on anatomic characteristics, shunt volume (Qp/Qs), and clinical symptoms. CT is increasingly used for pre- and post-interventional imaging in the setting of percutaneous ASD closure (**Figure 13.2**).[175] Several papers describe 'septal pouch' as a blind ending tubular remnant at the interatrial septum.[176,177]

Ventricular septal defects (VSDs) are common in childhood, but either closed spontaneously or are closed surgically at an early age. Therefore, in adult populations, mainly surgical changes are identified. The different types of VSD (perimembranous VSD, muscular or -apical VSD, inlet of atrioventricular canal VSD, supracristal or sub-aortic VSD) are related to the embryonal development of the interventricular septum. CT can identify the defect and describe the relationship to surrounding structures (**Figures 13.3–13.5**). Echocardiography, MRI, and cardiac catheterization with evaluation of oxygen saturation, flow, shunt volume (Qp/Qs), and pressure measurements are important for functional assessment.

Arrhythmogenic right ventricular dysplasia (ARVD), LV non-compaction, and hypertrophic obstructive cardiomyopathy (HOCM) are described in Chapter 4.

DOI: 10.1201/9781003153641-15

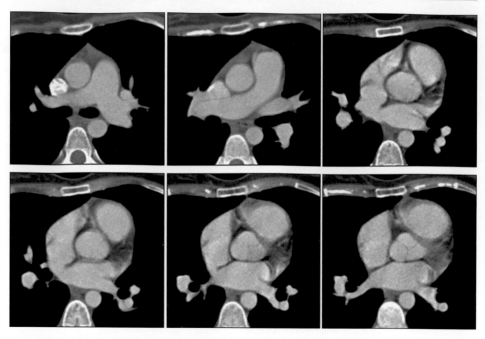

Figure 13.1 Sinus venosus atrial septal defect (ASD). This figure shows images of a sinus venosus type atrial septal defect. The defect is located at the roof of the intraatrial septum. There is partial anomalous venous return involving the superior right pulmonary vein, which empties into the superior vena cava (middle upper panel).

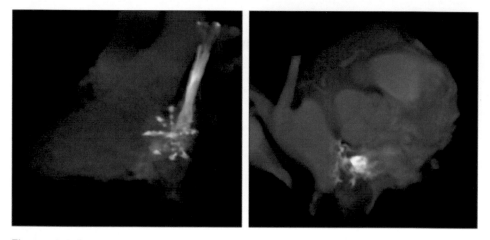

Figure 13.2 Percutaneous atrial septal defect (ASD) closure. CT is used for pre- and post-interventional imaging in the setting of percutaneous closure. This figure shows post-interventional images after PFO closure with a #33 Cardio-seal device. The cardiac structures are faded in this VRI image. The high-density metal struts are clearly seen in relation to the surrounding structures.

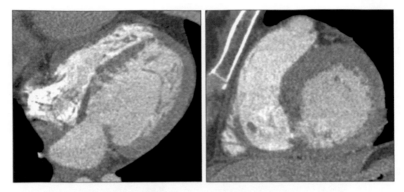

Figure 13.3 Ventricular septal defect. These images show a small left ventricular septal defect in the inferior aspect of the basal septum.

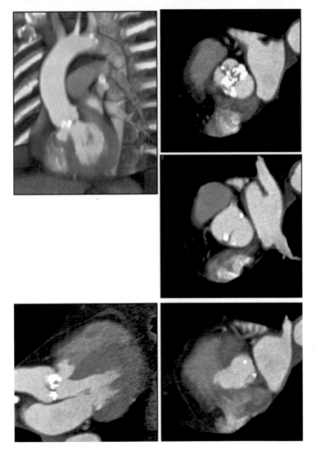

Figure 13.4 Aneurysm of membranous interventricular septum. This figure shows images of an example of an aneurysm of the membranous interventricular septum (windsock aneurysm). Below the right leaflet of the aortic valve, there is a small saccular outpouching of the membranous interventricular septum, extending to the right ventricle. The left upper panel shows a VRI image of the aortic root with the aneurysm visible inferior to the right coronary cups. The left lower panel shows the aneurysm anterior to the left ventricular outflow tract in a three-chamber view. The right lower panel shows a short-axis view of the aortic root at the level of the aneurysm. The aneurysm leads to eccentric outpouching (7 o'clock). Additional short-axis views at higher levels show a densely calcified bicuspid aortic valve (right middle panel).

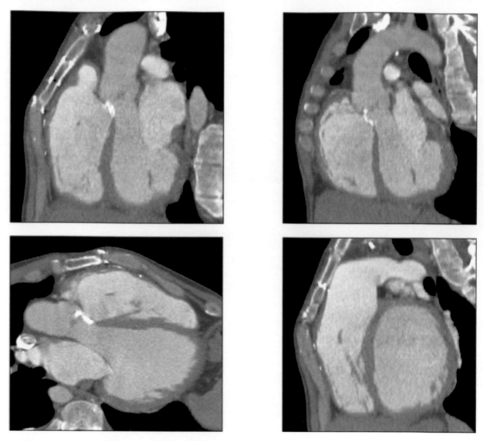

Figure 13.5 Surgically repaired VSD in tetralogy of Fallot. This figure shows images of a patient with repaired tetralogy of Fallot. There is dilatation of both ventricles. The patient has undergone reconstruction of the pulmonary outflow tract and closure of the ventricular septal defect with a patch.

13.2 Pericardial Disease

Images of patients with absence of the pericardium (**Figures 5.2** and **5.3**) are shown in Chapter 5.

13.3 Valvular Heart Disease

Images of patients with bicuspid and quatrocuspid aortic valves (**Figures 6.1–6.3**), sub-aortic membrane (**Figure 6.5**), and Ebstein's anomaly of the tricuspid valve (**Figure 6.11**) are included in Chapter 6.

13.4 Coronary Arteries

The assessment of coronary anomalies is a strength of MDCT. Image reconstruction allows definition of the origin and course of anomalous arteries.

There are multiple different types of anomalies with different clinical significance.[178] Variants without clinical significance include those with a course of the anomalous vessel between the root and adjacent low pressure chambers (LA, RA), e.g. an RCA origin of the non-coronary instead of the right coronary cusp. More significant is the origin of the right or left coronary system from the contralateral cusp or artery with course between aorta and pulmonary artery (PA) (**Figures 13.6** and **13.7**). The course of the anomalous artery relative to the aorta and PA determines the clinical significance. A course of the anomalous artery posterior to the aortic root, between the aortic root and the left atrium (**Figure 13.8**), is considered a benign course, because the left atrium is a low-pressure chamber. In contrast, a course of the anomalous artery anterior to the aortic root, between the aorta and the PA, can be associated with intermittent compression between the two high pressure vessels. For this 'inter-arterial' course, two variants are described: (1) a low course, crossing between the aortic root and pulmonary outflow, extending into the interventricular septum, is described as intracristal (**Figures 13.9–13.11**). Some investigators describe that the risk of compression with significant clinical complications for this variant is lower. (2) In contrast, a high course, crossing between the aorta and the PA, has a higher risk of systolic compression between the two structures (**Figures 13.12** and **13.13**). The demonstration of an anomalous course between the aorta and the PA may therefore define an indication of surgical correction. However, clinical data demonstrates that clinical symptoms and documentation of myocardial ischemia are most critical in the decision about management in these patients.[179,180] An advantage of CT is description

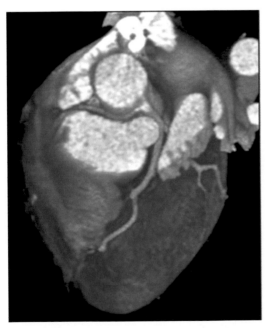
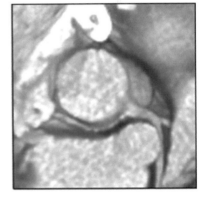

Figure 13.6 Anomalous origin of RCA from LM. This figure shows images of a 15-year-old patient, symptomatic with exertional chest pain. The right coronary artery originates from the left main coronary artery. The RCA takes a course between the right ventricular outflow tract and the aorta and continues in the right atrioventricular groove.

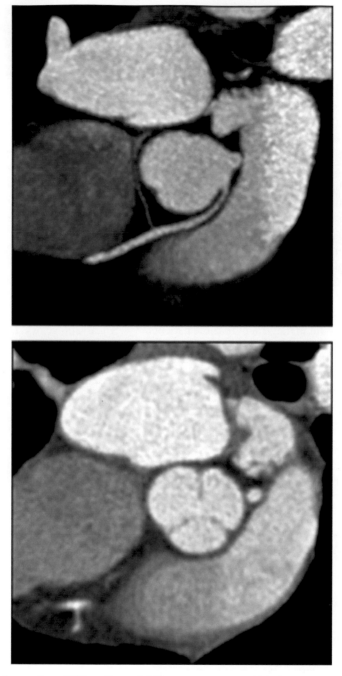

Figure 13.7 Anomalous RCA ostium of left coronary cusp. This figure shows images of an anomalous RCA. The RCA has a separate ostium from the left cusp, originating towards the raphe between the left and right coronary cusp. The RCA takes a course between the pulmonary outflow tract/pulmonary artery (at the level of the pulmonary valve) and aorta into the right atrioventricular groove.

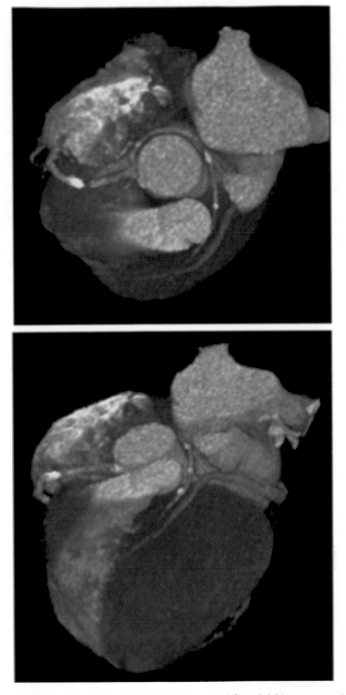

Figure 13.8 Anomalous coronary origin. In this figure, the left and right coronary arteries originate with a common coronary ostium from the right coronary cusp. The left coronary artery then takes a course posterior to aortic root, between the aortic root and the left atrium. Because the left atrium is a low-pressure system, this anomaly has low risk of complication.

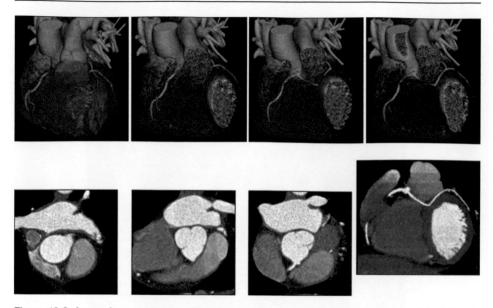

Figure 13.9 Anomalous coronary artery, intraseptal course (1). Anomalous origin of the left main coronary artery from the right coronary cusp, with a common ostium together with the right coronary artery. The left main takes an inferior, intramyocardial course below the level of the pulmonic valve in the interventricular septum between the left and right ventricular outflow tract. The vessel resurfaces on the anterior aspect of the left ventricle and trifurcates into the LAD, a Ramus intermedius, and the left circumflex.

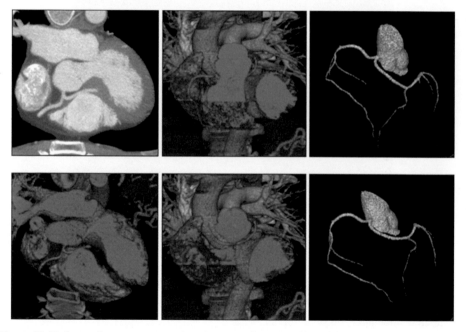

Figure 13.10 Anomalous coronary artery, intraseptal course (2). Another patient with an anomalous origin of the left main coronary artery with a common ostium from the right coronary cusp is shown in these images. The volume-rendered images show the low course of the anomalous left main with the typical 'hammock' appearance. The MIP image (left upper panel) shows the associated position of the left main in the interventricular septum. The vessel resurfaces on the anterior aspect of the left ventricle.

180

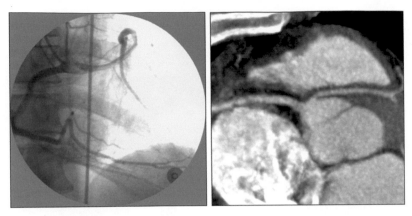

Figure 13.11 Anomalous coronary artery, comparison of angiography and CT. Images of a patient with suspected anomaly of the left coronary system. The angiogram shows the origin of the LAD and RCA from a common ostium in the right coronary cusp. This figure compares angiographic and CT images. The CT demonstrates the origin of the left coronary system from the right coronary sinus of Valsalva. There is a common ostium shared by the left coronary system and the RCA. The anomalous LM coronary artery takes a course between the aortic root and the outflow tract of the right ventricle within the musculature of the crista of the upper interventricular septum.

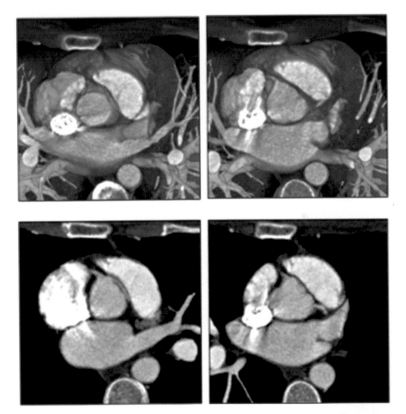

Figure 13.12 Anomalous coronary artery, course between aorta and pulmonary artery (1). Similar to the previous figure, the LAD originates from the right coronary cusp and takes a course anterior to the aortic root. However, the LAD crosses above the level of the pulmonary artery, between the aorta and pulmonary artery. This anatomy is associated with a higher risk of systolic compression and clinical complications.

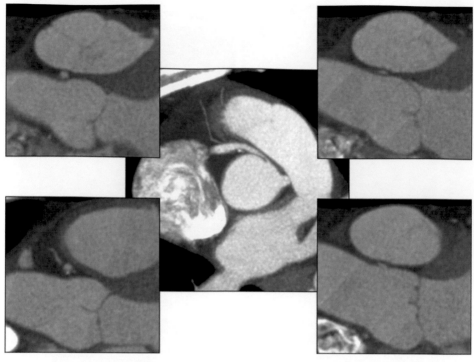

Figure 13.13 Anomalous coronary artery, course between aorta and pulmonary artery (2).
This figure shows images of a symptomatic patient with an anomalous RCA. The RCA originates from the left coronary cusp, next to the left main ostium and takes an initial course between the pulmonary artery and aorta (centre panel). There is slit-like compression of the artery at the ostium and the proximal interarterial course (right panels). More distally, the RCA has a normal diameter (left upper panel), but shows eccentric, partially calcified atherosclerotic plaque accumulation (centre and left lower panels).

of the relationship of the anomalous coronary artery to other cardiovascular structures. This becomes obvious in cases of coronary fistulas (**Figures 13.14–13.17**) and in the evaluation of an intramyocardial course of a coronary muscle bridge (**Figures 13.18 and 13.19**).

The large branches of the coronary arteries are located in the epicardial fat. However, individual segments occasionally have an intramyocardial location (myocardial bridges). MDCT permits the evaluation of these segments. CT is likely very sensitive in the identification of bridges but does not provide information about the hemodynamic significance of bridges. In contrast, conventional angiography, which defines bridges by their systolic compression, is likely more specific for significant myocardial bridges.

13.5 Pulmonary Veins

Partial anomalous return of the pulmonary veins is seen as an isolated finding or as part of other abnormalities (**Figures 13.20** and **13.21**).

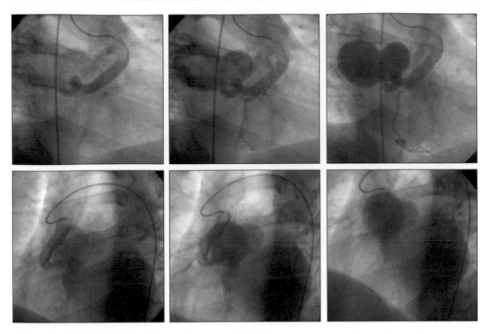

Figure 13.14 Coronary fistula, angiogram. This figure shows images of a patient with a complex coronary fistula. The fistula originates in the right coronary sinus. It gives rise to the RCA and then continues into a bell-shaped structure, which eventually connects to the left atrium.

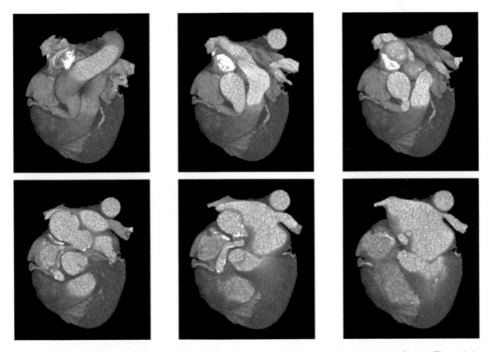

Figure 13.15 Coronary fistula, CT. Corresponding CT images are shown in this figure. The origin of the fistula of the right coronary cusp is seen (left upper panel). The other panels show cut planes at different levels. The origin of the right coronary artery (RCA) and the connection of the fistula to the bell-shaped structure are demonstrated.

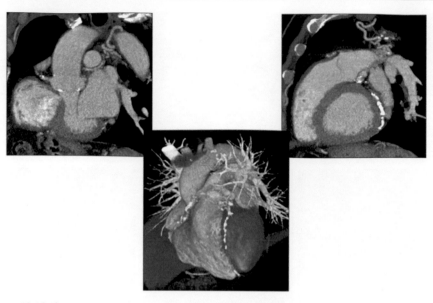

Figure 13.16 Coronary arteriovenous malformation (AVM) with connection to pulmonary artery (1). This and the next figure show an arteriovenous malformation with contributions from the conus branch of the right coronary artery as well as left main and left anterior descending coronary artery. There appears to be an additional supply from a branch of the left internal mammary artery although this is incompletely imaged. The malformation appears to drain into the pulmonary artery just above the pulmonary valve. There is coronary artery atherosclerosis involving the coronary arteries.

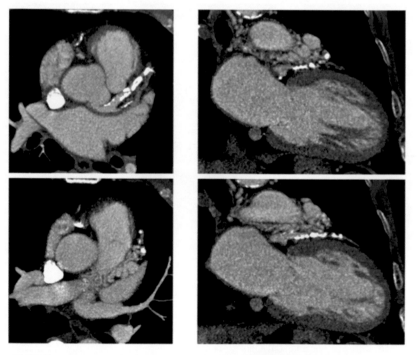

Figure 13.17 Coronary arteriovenous malformation (AVM) with connection to pulmonary artery (2). The images in this figure demonstrate the vessel tangle located between the proximal left anterior descending coronary artery and pulmonary artery.

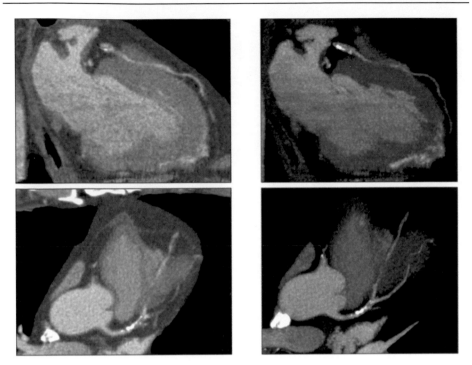

Figure 13.18 Myocardial bridge (1). CT is likely very sensitive in the identification of bridges but does not provide information about the hemodynamic significance of bridges. An example is shown in this figure. The proximal LAD has a brief intramyocardial course consistent with a myocardial bridge. There are calcified atherosclerotic changes in the proximal LAD. Typically, the intramyocardial segment is spared.

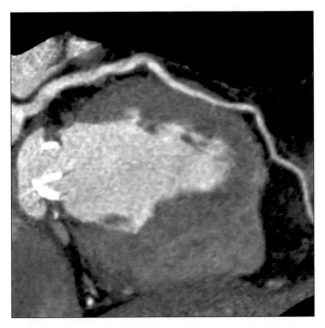

Figure 13.19 Myocardial bridge (2). Another example is shown in this figure. The mid-LAD has a shallow intramyocardial course consistent with a myocardial bridge.

185

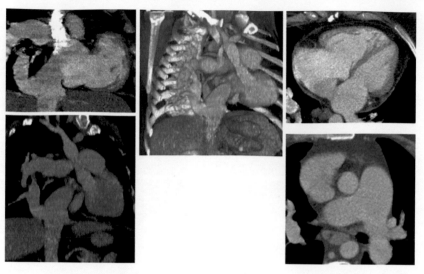

Figure 13.20 Partial anomalous return of pulmonary veins (Scimitar syndrome). Partial anomalous return of the pulmonary veins is seen as an isolated finding or as part of other abnormalities. In this patient, there is anomalous pulmonary venous return of the right pulmonary veins to the inferior vena cava above the diaphragm. Together with hypoplasia of the right lung lobe, that finding is consistent with the Scimitar syndrome. There is normal central venous return. The cardiac chambers are notable for moderate to severe right atrial and right ventricular enlargement. There is severe dilatation of the central pulmonary artery, measuring 4.6 cm before the bifurcation (right lower panel).

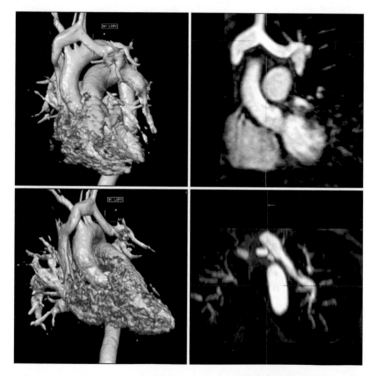

Figure 13.21 Partial anomalous return of the left superior pulmonary vein. This figure shows images of a left superior pulmonary vein, draining into the left subclavian vein.

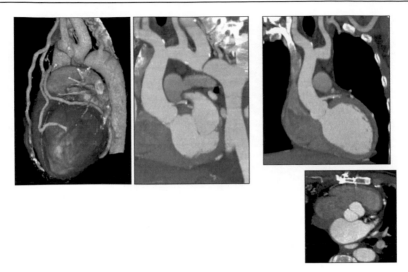

Figure 13.22 **Aortic coarctation.** This figure shows images of a patient with a remote history of coronary bypass surgery. The CT scan demonstrates aortic coarctation. There is hypoplasia of the arch with discrete juxtaductal narrowing of the isthmus. There are prominent collaterals including the internal mammary arteries. The known association with bicuspid aortic valve should be considered (right lower panel).

13.6 Aortic Disease

CT can demonstrate the anatomy of unrepaired aortic coarctation (**Figures 13.22** and **13.23**), and results after percutaneous endovascular (**Figures 13.24** and **13.25**) and surgical (**Figures 13.26** and **13.27**) repair. The known association with the bicuspid aortic valve should be considered (**Figure 13.22**).

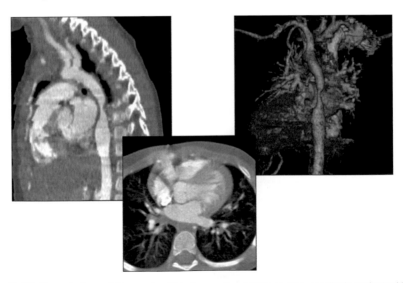

Figure 13.23 **Coarctation of the aorta.** This figure shows images of a paediatric patient with aortic coarctation. Because of the young age of the patient, the scan was performed with the patient breathing and without ECG gating. Despite the resulting decrease in image quality, the images are diagnostic. However, radiation exposure in paediatric patients requires careful consideration of indication and alternative imaging modalities.

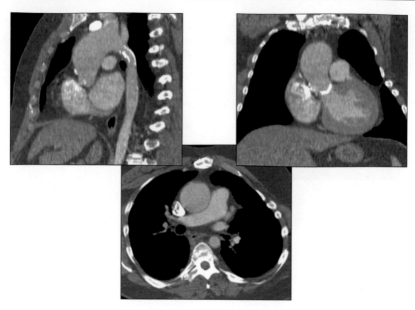

Figure 13.24 Coarctation and stent. This figure shows images of a patient with a history of aortic coarctation and percutaneous repair with a stent. There is replacement of the aortic valve with a low-profile mechanical prosthesis (right upper panel). There is fusiform dilatation of the mid-ascending aorta with a maximum diameter of 5.3 cm. Beyond the origin of the left subclavian artery, there is rapid tapering of the isthmus to approximately 1.5 cm. An intact stent covering the area of the coarctation is seen.

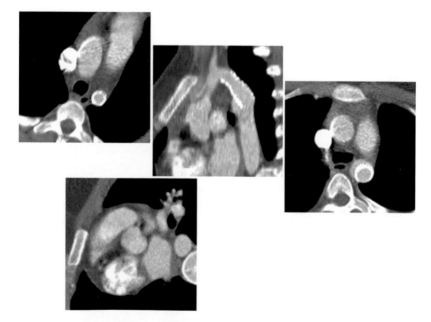

Figure 13.25 Coarctation of the aorta/stent. This figure shows images of a patient with a history of aortic coarctation, status post-remote surgical repair with a subclavian flap and subsequent stent placement for residual stenosis. The aortic valve appears bicuspid (left lower panel), with fusion of the left and right coronary cusps. The aortic root has normal dimensions. There is a stent in the area of the proximal descending aorta. Minimal stent diameter in the proximal segment is 1.5 cm. At the distal end, the stent is not completely apposed to the aortic wall. In this segment, the native aorta measures 2.5 cm.

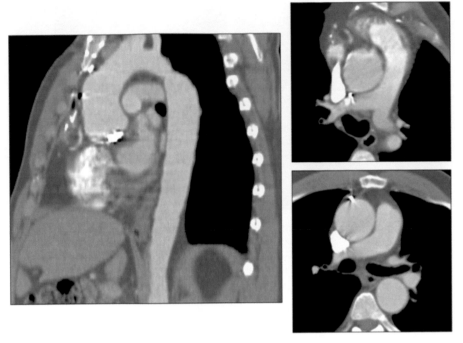

Figure 13.26 Coarctation and surgical repair (1). This figure shows images of a patient with a history of surgical repair of aortic coarctation and aortic valve repair. There is evidence of end-to-end anastomosis of the aorta.

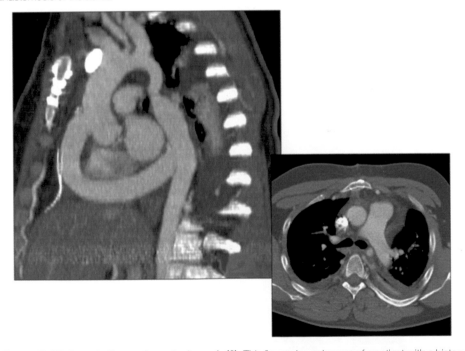

Figure 13.27 Coarctation and surgical repair (2). This figure shows images of a patient with a history of surgical repair of aortic coarctation. There is a shunt graft extending from the ascending to descending thoracic aorta. The narrowed area of the proximal descending aorta is seen.

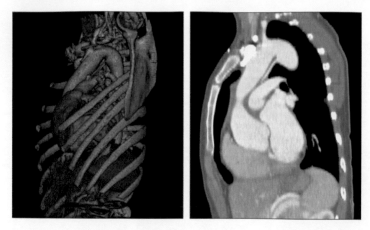

Figure 13.28 Patent ductus arteriosus (PDA). The ductus arteriosus (PDA) is a communication between the descending aorta (beyond left subclavian) and main pulmonary artery (near bifurcation) and physiologically bypasses the pulmonary circulation in the fetus. A patent ductus can be found in asymptomatic adults, in particular if the size is small.

Marfan syndrome, a multisystem connective-tissue disorder associated with a mutation in the fibrillin (*FBN1*) gene, Ehlers-Danlos syndrome, and Loeye-Dietz syndrome are associated with aortic disease (see Chapter 9).

13.7 Arteriovenous Shunt Defects

The ductus arteriosus is a communication between the proximal descending aorta and main PA. In the fetus, it physiologically bypasses the pulmonary circulation. A patent ductus can be found in asymptomatic adults, in particular if the size is small (**Figures 13.28–13.30**). The fibrotic and often calcified remnant is called the ligamentum arteriosum (**Figure 13.30**).

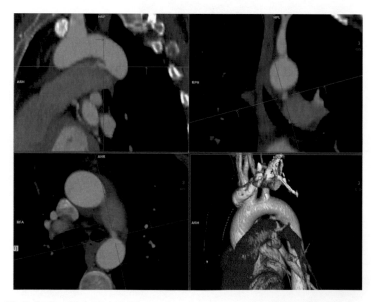

Figure 13.29 Ductus arteriosus. This figure shows another example of a small patent ductus arteriosis.

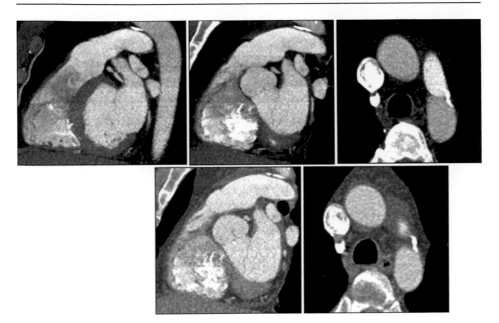

Figure 13.30 Spontaneous closure of ductus arteriosus: Ligamentum arteriosum.
Physiologically, the ductus arteriosus closes after birth. The fibrotic remnant of the ductus arteriosus is called the ligamentum arteriosum.

References

1. Ambrose J, Hounsfield G. Computerized transverse axial tomography. Br J Radiol. 1973;46:148–149.
2. Hounsfield GN. Computed medical imaging. Science. 1980;210:22–28.
3. Brenner DJ, Hall EJ. Computed tomography – an increasing source of radiation exposure. N Engl J Med. 2007;357:2277–2284.
4. Schoenhagen P, Numburi U, Halliburton SS, Aulbach P, von Roden M, Desai MY, Rodriguez LL, Kapadia SR, Tuzcu EM, Lytle BW. Three-dimensional imaging in the context of minimally invasive and transcatheter cardiovascular interventions using multidetector computed tomography: from pre-operative planning to intra-operative guidance. Eur Heart J. 2010;31:2727–2740.
5. Dewey M. Cardiac CT, 2nd ed. Springer, 2014. ISBN 978-3-642-41882-2.
6. Budoff MJ, Raggi P. Coronary artery disease progression assessed by electron-beam computed tomography. Am J Cardiol. 2001;88:46E–50E.
7. Kalendar WA, Seissler W, Klotz E, Vock P. Spiral volumetric CT with single-breath-hold technique, continuous transport, and continuous scanner rotation. Radiology. 1990;176:181–183.
8. Klingenbeck-Regn K, Schaller S, Flohr T, Ohnesorge B, Kopp A, Baum U. Subsecond multi-slice computed tomography: basics and applications. Eur J Radiol. 1999;31:110–124.
9. Flohr TG, McCollough CH, Bruder H, Petersilka M, Gruber K, Suss C, Grasruck M, Stierstorfer K, Krauss B, Raupach R, Primak AN, Kuttner A, Achenbach S, Becker C, Kopp A, Ohnesorge BM. First performance evaluation of a dual-source CT (DSCT) system. Eur Radiol. 2006;16:256–268.
10. Blank M, Kalendar WA. Medical volume exploration: gaining insights virtually. Eur J Radiol. 2000;33:161–169.
11. Rubin GD, Beaulieu CF, Argiro V, et al. Perspective volume rendering of CT and MR images: applications for endoscopic imaging. Radiology. 1996;199:321–330.
12. Mahnken AH, Muhlenbruch G, Koos R, et al. Automated vs. manual assessment of left ventricular function in cardiac multidetector row computed tomography: comparison with magnetic resonance imaging. Eur Radiol. 2006;16:1416–1423.
13. Hong C, Becker CR, Huber A, et al. ECG-gated reconstructed multidetector row CT coronary angiography: effect of varying trigger delay on image quality. Radiology. 2001;220:712–717.
14. Kopp AF, Schroeder S, Kuettner A, et al. Coronary arteries: retrospectively ECG-gated multidetector row CT angiography with selective optimization of the image reconstruction window. Radiology. 2001;221:683–688.
15. Hsieh, J, Section 6.4 in Computed Tomography: Principles, Design, Artifacts, and Recent Advance, 2nd ed. SPIE Press.
16. Halliburton SS, Abbara S, Chen MY, et al. SCCT guidelines on radiation dose and dose-optimization strategies in cardiovascular CT. J Cardiovasc Comput Tomogr. 2011;5(4):198–224.
17. Ohnesorge B, Flohr T, Becker C, et al. Cardiac imaging by means of electrocardiographically gated multisection spiral CT: initial experience. Radiology. 2000;217:564–571.

18. Lell M, Marwan M, Schepis T, Pflederer T, Anders K, Flohr T, Allmendinger T, Kalender W, Ertel D, Thierfelder C, Kuettner A, Ropers D, Daniel WG, Achenbach S. Prospectively ECG-triggered high-pitch spiral acquisition for coronary CT angiography using dualsource CT: technique and initial experience. Eur Radiol. 2009;19:2576–2583.

19. Jakobs T, Becker CR, Ohnesorge B, et al. Multislice helical CT of the heart with retrospective ECG gating: reduction of radiation exposure by ECG-controlled tube current modulation. Eur Radiol. 2002;12:1081–1086.

20. Flohr T, Ohnesorge B. Heart rate adaptive optimization of spatial and temporal resolution for electrocardiogram-gated multislice spiral CT of the heart. J Computer Assist Tomogr. 2001;25:907–923.

21. Stierstorfer K, Flohr T, Bruder H. Segmented multiple plane reconstruction: a novel approximate reconstruction scheme for multi-slice spiral CT. Phys Med Biol. 2002;47:2571–2581.

22. Boese JM, Bahner ML, Albers J, van Kaick G. Optimizing temporal resolution in CT with retrospective ECG gating. Radiologe. 2000;40:123–129.

23. Willemink MJ, Persson M, Pourmorteza A, Pelc NJ, Fleischmann D. Photon-counting CT: technical principles and clinical prospects. Radiology. 2018;289(2):293–312.

24. Zipes DP, Libby P, Bonow RO, Mann DL, Tomaselli GF. Braunwald's Heart Disease: A Textbook of Cardiovascular Medicine, 11th ed. Elsevier. ISBN-10: 0323462995, ISBN-13: 978-0323462990

25. Taylor AJ, Cerqueira M, Hodgson JM, et al. ACCF/SCCT/ACR/AHA/ASE/ASNC/NASCI/SCAI/SCMR 2010 Appropriate Use Criteria for Cardiac Computed Tomography. Circulation. 2010;122:e525–e555; J Am Coll Cardiol. 2010;56:1864–1894; J Cardiovasc Comput Tomogr. 2010;4:407.e1–e33.

26. Doherty JU, Kort S, Mehran R, et al. ACC/AATS/AHA/ASE/ASNC/HRS/SCAI/SCCT/SCMR/STS 2019 Appropriate Use Criteria for Multimodality Imaging in the Assessment of Cardiac Structure and Function in Nonvalvular Heart Disease: A Report of the American College of Cardiology Appropriate Use Criteria Task Force, American Association for Thoracic Surgery, American Heart Association, American Society of Echocardiography, American Society of Nuclear Cardiology, Heart Rhythm Society, Society for Cardiovascular Angiography and Interventions, Society of Cardiovascular Computed Tomography, Society for Cardiovascular Magnetic Resonance, and the Society of Thoracic Surgeons. J Am Coll Cardiol. 2019;73(4):488–516.

27. Doherty JU, Kort S, Mehran R, Schoenhagen P, Soman P. J ACC/AATS/AHA/ASE/ASNC/HRS/SCAI/SCCT/SCMR/STS 2017 Appropriate Use Criteria for Multimodality Imaging in Valvular Heart Disease: A Report of the American College of Cardiology Appropriate Use Criteria Task Force, American Association for Thoracic Surgery, American Heart Association, American Society of Echocardiography, American Society of Nuclear Cardiology, Heart Rhythm Society, Society for Cardiovascular Angiography and Interventions, Society of Cardiovascular Computed Tomography, Society for Cardiovascular Magnetic Resonance, and Society of Thoracic Surgeons. J Am Coll Cardiol. 2017;70(13):1647–1672. Epub 2017 Sep 1.

28. François CJ, Schiebler ML, Reeder SB. Cardiac MRI evaluation of nonischemic cardiomyopathies. J Magn Reson Imaging. 2010;31:518–530.

29. Andreini D, Pontone G, Pepi M, et al. Diagnostic accuracy of multidetector computed tomography coronary angiography in patients with dilated cardiomyopathy. J Am Coll Cardiol. 2007;49:2044–2050.

30. Oechslin EN, Attenhofer Jost CH, Rojas JR, Kaufmann PA, Jenni R. Long-term follow-up of 34 adults with isolated left ventricular noncompaction: a distinct cardiomyopathy with poor prognosis. J Am Coll Cardiol. 2000;36:493–500.

31. Jenni R, Oechslin E, Schneider J, Attenhofer Jost C, Kaufmann PA. Echocardiographic and pathoanatomical characteristics of isolated left ventricular non-compaction: a step towards classification as a distinct cardiomyopathy. Heart. 2001;86:666–671.

32. Petersen SE, Selvanayagam JB, Wiesmann F, et al. Left ventricular non-compaction: insights from cardiovascular magnetic resonance imaging. J Am Coll Cardiol. 2005;46:101–105.

33. Pignatelli RH, McMahon CJ, Dreyer WJ, et al. Clinical characterization of left ventricular noncompaction in children: a relatively common form of cardiomyopathy. Circulation. 2003;108:2672–2678.

34. Melendez-Ramirez G, Castillo-Castellon F, Espinola-Zavaleta N, Meave A, Kimura-Hayama ET. Left ventricular noncompaction: a proposal of new diagnostic criteria by multidetector computed tomography. J Cardiovasc Comput Tomogr. 2012;6:346–354.

35. Sengupta PP, Mohan JC, Mehta V, et al. Comparison of echocardiographic features of noncompaction of the left ventricle in adults versus idiopathic dilated cardiomyopathy in adults. Am J Cardiol. 2004;94:389–391.

36. Kohli SK, Pantazis AA, Shah JS, et al. Diagnosis of left-ventricular non-compaction in patients with left-ventricular systolic dysfunction: time for a reappraisal of diagnostic criteria? Eur Heart J. 2008;29:89–95.

37. Kawel N, Nacif M, Arai AE, et al. Trabeculated (noncompacted) and compact myocardium in adults: the multi-ethnic study of atherosclerosis. Circ Cardiovasc Imaging. 2012;5:357–366.

38. Nagueh SF, Bierig SM, Budoff MJ, et al. American Society of Echocardiography clinical recommendations for multimodality cardiovascular imaging of patients with hypertrophic cardiomyopathy: J Am Soc Echocardiogr. 2011;24:473–498.

39. Kwon DH, Smedira NG, Rodriguez ER, et al. Cardiac magnetic resonance detection of myocardial scarring in hypertrophic cardiomyopathy: correlation with histopathology and prevalence of ventricular tachycardia. J Am Coll Cardiol. 2009;54:242–249.

40. Zhao L, Ma X, Delano MC, et al. Assessment of myocardial fibrosis and coronary arteries in hypertrophic cardiomyopathy using combined arterial and delayed enhanced CT: comparison with MR and coronary angiography. Eur Radiol. 2013;23:1034–1043.

41. Raymond Y. Kwong, MD; Rodney H. Falk, MD. Cardiovascular Magnetic Resonance in Cardiac Amyloidosis. Circulation. 2005;111:122–124.

42. Hulot JS, Jouven X, Empana JP, Frank R, Fontaine G. Natural history and risk stratification of arrhythmogenic right ventricular dysplasia/cardiomyopathy. Circulation. 2004;110:1879–1884.

43. Marcus FI, McKenna WJ, Sherrill D, et al. Diagnosis of arrhythmogenic right ventricular cardiomyopathy/dysplasia: proposed modification of the Task Force Criteria. Eur Heart J. 2010;31:806–814.

44. Nieman K, Cury RC, Ferencik M, et al. Differentiation of recent and chronic myocardial infarction by cardiac computed tomography. Am J Cardiol. 2006;98:303–308.

45. Ortiz-Pérez JT, Lee DC, Meyers SN, Davidson CJ, Bonow RO, Wu E. Determinants of myocardial salvage during acute myocardial infarction: evaluation with a combined angiographic and CMR myocardial salvage index. JACC Cardiovasc Imaging. 2010;3:491–500.

46. Wright J, Adriaenssens T, Dymarkowski S, Desmet W, Bogaert J. Quantification of myocardial area at risk with T2-weighted CMR: comparison with contrast-enhanced CMR and coronary angiography. JACC Cardiovasc Imaging. 2009;2:825–831.

47. Berry C, Kellman P, Mancini C, et al. Magnetic resonance imaging delineates the ischemic area at risk and myocardial salvage in patients with acute myocardial infarction. Circ Cardiovasc Imaging. 2010;3:527–535.

48. Wong DT, Richardson JD, Puri R, et al. The role of cardiac magnetic resonance imaging following acute myocardial infarction. Eur Radiol. 2012;22(8):1757–1768.

49. Baks T, Cademartiri F, Moelker AD, et al. Multislice computed tomography and magnetic resonance imaging for the assessment of reperfused acute myocardial infarction. J Am Coll Cardiol. 2006;48:144–152.

50. Rodriguez-Granillo GA, Rosales MA, Baum S, et al. Early assessment of myocardial viability by the use of delayed enhancement computed tomography after primary percutaneous coronary intervention. JACC Cardiovasc Imaging. 2009;2:1072–1081.

51. Hoffmann U, Truong QA, Schoenfeld DA, et al; ROMICAT-II Investigators. Coronary CT angiography versus standard evaluation in acute chest pain. N Engl J Med. 2012;367:299–308.

52. Hoffmann U, Bamberg F, Chae CU, et al. Coronary computed tomography angiography for early triage of patients with acute chest pain: the ROMICAT (Rule Out Myocardial Infarction using Computer Assisted Tomography) trial. J Am Coll Cardiol. 2009;53:1642–1650.

53. Goldstein JA, Chinnaiyan KM, Abidov A, et al; CT-STAT Investigators. The CT-STAT (Coronary Computed Tomographic Angiography for Systematic Triage of Acute Chest Pain Patients to Treatment) trial. J Am Coll Cardiol. 2011;58:1414–1422.

54. Litt HI, Gatsonis C, Snyder B, et al. CT angiography for safe discharge of patients with possible acute coronary syndromes. N Engl J Med. 2012;366:1393–1403.

55. Twerenbold R, Boeddinghaus J, Nestelberger T, Wildi K, Rubini Gimenez M, Badertscher P, Mueller clinical use of high-sensitivity cardiac troponin in patients with suspected myocardial infarction. J Am Coll Cardiol. 2017;70(8):996–1012.

56. Paul JF, Macé L, Caussin C, et al. Multirow detector computed tomography assessment of intraseptal dissection and ventricular pseudoaneurysm in postinfarction ventricular septal defect. Circulation. 2001;104:497–498.

57. Friedrich MG, Sechtem U, Schulz-Menger J, et al; International Consensus Group on Cardiovascular Magnetic Resonance in Myocarditis. A JACC White Paper. J Am Coll Cardiol. 2009;53(17):1475–1487.

58. Brouwer WP, Germans T, Head MC, et al. Multiple myocardial crypts on modified long-axis view are a specific finding in pre-hypertrophic HCM mutation carriers. Eur Heart J Cardiovasc Imaging. 2012;13(4):292–297.

59. Child N, Muhr T, Sammut E, et al. Prevalence of myocardial crypts in a large retrospective cohort study by cardiovascular magnetic resonance. J Cardiovasc Magn Reson. 2014 ;16(1):66.

60. Kim YY, Klein AL, Halliburton SS, et al. Left atrial appendage filling defects identified by multidetector computed tomography in patients undergoing radiofrequency pulmonary vein antral isolation: a comparison with transesophageal echocardiography. Am Heart J. 2007;154:1199–1205.

61. Krauser DG, Cham MD, Tortolani AJ, et al. Clinical utility of delayed-contrast computed tomography for tissue characterization of cardiac thrombus. J Cardiovasc Comput Tomogr. 2007;1(2):114–118.

62. Heyer CM, Kagel T, Lemburg SP, Bauer TT, Nicolas V. Lipomatous hypertrophy of the interatrial septum: a prospective study of incidence, imaging findings, and clinical symptoms. Chest. 2003;124:2068–2073.

63. Meaney JF, Kazerooni EA, Jamadar DA, Korobkin M. CT appearance of lipomatous hypertrophy of the interatrial septum. AJR Am J Roentgenol. 1997;168:1081–1084.

64. Klein AL, Abbara S, Agler DA, et al. American Society of Echocardiography clinical recommendations for multimodality cardiovascular imaging of patients with pericardial disease: endorsed by the Society for Cardiovascular Magnetic Resonance and Society of Cardiovascular Computed Tomography. J Am Soc Echocardiogr. 2013;26:965–1012.

65. Taylor AM, Dymarkowski S, Verbeken EK, Bogaert J. Detection of pericardial inflammation with late-enhancement cardiac magnetic resonance imaging: initial results. Eur Radiol. 2006;16:569–574.

66. Zurick AO, Bolen MA, Kwon DH, et al. Pericardial delayed hyperenhancement with CMR imaging in patients with constrictive pericarditis undergoing surgical pericardiectomy: a case series with histopathological correlation. JACC Cardiovasc Imaging. 2011;4:1180–1191.

67. Feng D, Glockner J, Kim K, et al. Cardiac magnetic resonance imaging pericardial late gadolinium enhancement and elevated inflammatory markers can predict the reversibility of constrictive pericarditis after antiinflammatory medical therapy: a pilot study. Circulation. 2011;124:1830–1837.

68. Feuchtner GM, Dichtl W, Friedrich GJ, et al. Multislice computed tomography for detection of patients with aortic valve stenosis and quantification of severity. J Am Coll Cardiol. 2006;47:1410–1417.

69. Toh H, Mori S, Izawa Y, et al. Prevalence and extent of mitral annular disjunction in structurally normal hearts: comprehensive 3D analysis using cardiac computed tomography. Eur Heart J Cardiovasc Imaging. 2021:jeab022. Online ahead of print.

70. Wang TKM, Bin Saeedan M, Chan N, et al. Complementary diagnostic and prognostic contributions of cardiac computed tomography for infective endocarditis surgery. Circ Cardiovasc Imaging. 2020;13(9):e011126. Epub 2020 Sep 9.

71. Koneru S, Huang SS, Oldan J, et al. Role of preoperative cardiac CT in the evaluation of infective endocarditis: comparison with transesophageal echocardiography and surgical findings. Cardiovasc Diagn Ther. 2018;8(4):439–449.

72. Blanke P, Weir-McCall JR, Achenbach S, et al. Computed tomography imaging in the context of transcatheter aortic valve implantation (TAVI)/transcatheter aortic valve replacement (TAVR): an expert consensus document of the Society of Cardiovascular Computed Tomography. J Cardiovasc Comput Tomogr. 2019;13(1):1–20.

73. Lou J, Obuchowski NA, Krishnaswamy A, et al. Manual, semiautomated, and fully automated measurement of the aortic annulus for planning of transcatheter aortic valve replacement (TAVR/TAVI): analysis of interchangeability. J Cardiovasc Comput Tomogr. 2015;9(1):42–49.

74. Wuest W, Anders K, Schuhbaeck A, et al. Dual source multidetector CT-angiography before transcatheter aortic valve implantation (TAVI) using a high-pitch spiral acquisition mode. Eur Radiol. 2012;22(1):51–58.

75. Jabbour A, Ismail TF, Moat N, et al. Multimodality imaging in transcatheter aortic valve implantation and post-procedural aortic regurgitation: comparison among cardiovascular magnetic resonance, cardiac computed tomography, and echocardiography. J Am Coll Cardiol. 2011;58(21):2165–2173.

76. Jilaihawi H, Doctor N, Kashif M, et al. Aortic annular sizing for transcatheter aortic valve replacement using cross-sectional 3-dimensional transesophageal echocardiography. J Am Coll Cardiol. 2013:908–916.

77. Willson AB, Webb JG, Labounty TM, et al. 3-Dimensional aortic annular assessment by multidetector computed tomography predicts moderate or severe paravalvular regurgitation after transcatheter aortic valve replacement: a multicenter retrospective analysis. J Am Coll Cardiol. 2012;59(14):1287–1294.

78. Kurra V, Kapadia SR, Tuzcu EM, et al. Pre-procedural imaging of aortic root orientation and dimensions: comparison between X-ray angiographic planar imaging and 3-dimensional multidetector row computed tomography. JACC Cardiovasc Interv. 2010;3(1):105–113.

79. Makkar RR, Blanke P, Leipsic J, et al. Subclinical leaflet thrombosis in transcatheter and surgical bioprosthetic valves: PARTNER 3 cardiac computed tomography substudy. J Am Coll Cardiol. 2020;75(24):3003–3015.

80. Natarajan N, Patel P, Bartel T, et al. Peri-procedural imaging for transcatheter mitral valve replacement. Cardiovasc Diagn Ther. 2016;6(2):144–159.

81. Kapadia S, Krishnaswamy A, Layoun H, et al. Tricuspid annular dimensions in patients with severe mitral regurgitation without severe tricuspid regurgitation. Cardiovasc Diagn Ther. 2021;11(1):68–80.

82. Abbara S, Blanke P, Maroules CD, et al. SCCT guidelines for the performance and acquisition of coronary computed tomographic angiography: a report of the Society of Cardiovascular Computed Tomography Guidelines Committee: Endorsed by the North American Society for Cardiovascular Imaging (NASCI). J Cardiovasc Comput Tomogr. 2016;10(6):435–449.

83. Bastarrika G, Lee YS, Huda W, Ruzsics B, Costello P, Schoepf UJ. CT of coronary artery disease. Radiology. 2009;253(2):317–338.

84. Stone NJ, Robinson JG, Lichtenstein AH, et al. 2013 ACC/AHA guideline on the treatment of blood cholesterol to reduce atherosclerotic cardiovascular risk in adults: a report of the American College of Cardiology/American Heart Association Task Force on Practice Guidelines. Circulation. 2014;129(25 Suppl 2):S1–S45.

85. Libby P, Theroux P. Pathophysiology of coronary artery disease. Circulation. 2005;111:3481–3488.

86. Schmermund A, Erbel R. Unstable coronary plaque and its relation to coronary calcium. Circulation. 2001;104:1682–1687.

87. Agatston AS, Janowitz WR, Hildner FJ, Zusmer NR, Viamonte M, Detrano R. Quantification of coronary artery calcium using ultrafast computed tomography. J Am Coll Cardiol. 1990;15:827–832.

88. Ohnesorge B, Kopp AF, Fischbach R, et al. Reproducibility of coronary calcium quantification in repeat examinations with retrospectively ECG-gated multislice spiral CT. Eur Radiol. 2002;12:1532–1540.

89. Parikh P, Shah N, Ahmed H, Schoenhagen P, Fares M. Coronary artery calcium scoring: its practicality and clinical utility in primary care. Cleve Clin J Med. 2018;85(9):707–716.

90. Alashi A, Lang R, Seballos R, et al. Reclassification of coronary heart disease risk in a primary prevention setting: traditional risk factor assessment vs. coronary artery calcium scoring. Cardiovasc Diagn Ther. 2019;9(3):214–220.

91. Callister TQ, Raggi P, Cooil B, Lippolis NJ, Russo DJ. Effect of HMG-CoA reductase inhibitors on coronary artery disease by electron-beam computed tomography. N Engl J Med. 1998;339:1972–1978.

92. Achenbach S, Ropers D, Pohle K, et al. Influence of lipid-lowering therapy on the progression of coronary artery calcification. A prospective evaluation. Circulation. 2002;106:1077–1082.

93. Schoenhagen P, Tuzcu EM, Stillman AE, et al. Non-invasive assessment of plaque morphology and remodeling in mildly stenotic coronary segments: comparison of 16-slice computed tomography and intravascular ultrasound. Coron Artery Dis. 2003;14:459–462.

94. Achenbach S, Moselewski F, Ropers D, et al. Detection of calcified and noncalcified coronary atherosclerotic plaque by contrast-enhanced, submillimeter multidetector spiral computed tomography: a segment-based comparison with intravascular ultrasound. Circulation. 2004;109:14–17.

95. Schoenhagen P, Ziada KM, Kapadia SR, Crowe TD, Nissen SE, Tuzcu EM. Extent and direction of arterial remodeling in stable versus unstable coronary syndromes: an intravascular ultrasound study. Circulation. 2000;101:598–603.

96. Achenbach S, Ropers D, Hoffmann U, et al. Assessment of coronary remodeling in stenotic and nonstenotic coronary atherosclerotic lesions by multidetector spiral computed tomography. J Am Coll Cardiol. 2004;43:842–847.

97. Cury RC, Abbara S, Achenbach S, et al. J CAD-RADS™: Coronary Artery Disease – Reporting and Data System: An Expert Consensus Document of the Society of Cardiovascular Computed Tomography (SCCT), the American College of Radiology (ACR) and the North American Society for Cardiovascular Imaging (NASCI). Endorsed by the American College of Cardiology. J Am Coll Radiol. 2016;13(12 Pt A): 1458–1466.

98. Motoyama S, Kondo T, Sarai M, et al. Multislice computed tomographic characteristics of coronary lesions in acute coronary syndromes. J Am Coll Cardiol. 2007;50:319–326.

99. Motoyama S, Sarai M, Harigaya H, et al. Computed tomographic angiography characteristics of atherosclerotic plaques subsequently resulting in acute coronary syndrome. J Am Coll Cardiol. 2009;54:49–57.

100. Min JK, Shaw LJ, Devereux RB, et al. Prognostic value of multidetector coronary computed tomographic angiography for prediction of all-cause mortality. J Am Coll Cardiol. 2007;50:1161–1170.

101. Cho I, Chang HJ, Sung JM, et al; CONFIRM Investigators. Coronary computed tomographic angiography and risk of all-cause mortality and nonfatal myocardial infarction in subjects without chest pain syndrome from the CONFIRM Registry. Circulation. 2012;126:304–313.

102. Hulten EA, Carbonaro S, Petrillo SP, Mitchell JD, Villines TC. Prognostic value of cardiac computed tomography angiography: a systematic review and meta-analysis. J Am Coll Cardiol. 2011;57:1237–1247.

103. Lin FY, Shaw LJ, Dunning AM, et al. Mortality risk in symptomatic patients with nonobstructive coronary artery disease a prospective 2-center study of 2,583 patients undergoing 64-detector row coronary computed tomographic angiography. J Am Coll Cardiol. 2011;58(5):510–519.

104. Kopp AF, Schroeder S, Kuettner A, et al. Coronary arteries: retrospectively ECG-gated multidetector row CT angiography with selective optimization of the image reconstruction window. Radiology. 2001;221:683–688.

105. Raff GL, Abidov A, Achenbach S, et al; Society of Cardiovascular Computed Tomography. SCCT guidelines for the interpretation and reporting of coronary computed tomographic angiography. J Cardiovasc Comput Tomogr. 2009;3(2):122–136.

106. von Ballmoos MW, Haring B, Juillerat P, Alkadhi H. Meta-analysis: diagnostic performance of low-radiation-dose coronary computed tomography angiography. Ann Intern Med. 2011;154(6):413–420.

107. Mowatt G, Cook JA, Hillis GS, et al. 64-Slice computed tomography angiography in the diagnosis and assessment of coronary artery disease: systematic review and meta-analysis. Heart. 2008;94(11):1386–1393.

108. Meijboom WB, Meijs MF, Schuijf JD, et al. Diagnostic accuracy of 64-slice computed tomography coronary angiography: a prospective, multicenter, multivendor study. J Am Coll Cardiol. 2008;52:2135–2144.

109. Bamberg F, Sommer WH, Hoffmann V, et al. Meta-analysis and systematic review of the long-term predictive value of assessment of coronary atherosclerosis by contrast-enhanced coronary computed tomography angiography. J Am Coll Cardiol. 2011;57(24):2426–2436.

110. Min JK, Shaw LJ, Devereux RB, et al. Prognostic value of multidetector coronary computed tomographic angiography for prediction of all-cause mortality. J Am Coll Cardiol. 2007;50:1161–1170.

111. Kamdar AR, Meadows TA, Roselli EE, et al. Multidetector computed tomographic angiography in planning of reoperative cardiothoracic surgery. Ann Thorac Surg. 2008;85(4):1239–1245.

112. Kumbhani DJ, Ingelmo CP, Schoenhagen P, Curtin RJ, Flamm SD, Desai MY. Meta-analysis of diagnostic efficacy of 64-slice computed tomography in the evaluation of coronary in-stent restenosis. Am J Cardiol. 2009;103(12):1675–1681.

113. Yip A, Saw J. Spontaneous coronary artery dissection – a review. Cardiovasc Diagn Ther. 2015;5(1):37–48.

114. Alfonso F, Bastante T, Cuesta J, Rodríguez D, Benedicto A, Rivero F. Spontaneous coronary artery dissection: novel insights on diagnosis and management. Cardiovasc Diagn Ther. 2015;5(2):133–140.

115. Min JK, Leipsic J, Pencina MJ, et al. Diagnostic accuracy of fractional flow reserve from anatomic CT angiography. JAMA. 2012;308(12):1237–1245.

116. Nørgaard BL, Leipsic J, Gaur S, et al; NXT Trial Study Group. Diagnostic performance of noninvasive fractional flow reserve derived from coronary computed tomography angiography in suspected coronary artery disease: the NXT trial (Analysis of Coronary Blood Flow Using CT Angiography: Next Steps). J Am Coll Cardiol. 2014;63(12):1145–1155.

117. Blankstein R, Shturman LD, Rogers IS, et al. Adenosine-induced stress myocardial perfusion imaging using dual-source cardiac computed tomography. J Am Coll Cardiol. 2009;54:1072–1284.

118. Ho KT, Chua KC, Klotz E, Panknin C. Stress and rest dynamic myocardial perfusion imaging by evaluation of complete time-attenuation curves with dual-source CT. JACC Cardiovasc Imaging. 2010;3:811–820.

119. Rochitte CE, George RT, Chen MY, et al. Computed tomography angiography and perfusion to assess coronary artery stenosis causing perfusion defects by single photon emission computed tomography: the CORE320 study. Eur Heart J. 2014;35(17):1120–1130.

120. Ko BS, Wong DT, Nørgaard BL, et al. Diagnostic performance of transluminal attenuation gradient and noninvasive fractional flow reserve derived from 320-detector row CT angiography to diagnose hemodynamically significant coronary stenosis: an NXT substudy. Radiology. 2016;279(1):75–83.

121. Jongbloed MR, Lamb HJ, Bax JJ, et al. Noninvasive visualization of the cardiac venous system using multislice computed tomography. J Am Coll Cardiol. 2005;45:749–753.

122. Patel D, Sripariwuth A, Abozeed M, et al. Lead location as assessed on cardiac computed tomography and difficulty of percutaneous transvenous extraction. JACC Clin Electrophysiol. 2019;5(12):1432–1438.

123. Vedovati MC, Becattini C, Agnelli G, et al. Multidetector CT scan for acute pulmonary embolism: embolic burden and clinical outcome. Chest. 2012;142(6):1417–1424.

124. Saad EB, Marrouche NF, Saad CP, et al. Pulmonary vein stenosis after catheter ablation of atrial fibrillation: emergence of a new clinical syndromes. Ann Intern Med. 2003;138:634–638.

125. To AC, Gabriel RS, Park M, et al. Role of Transesophageal Echocardiography Compared to Computed Tomography in Evaluation of Pulmonary Vein Ablation for Atrial Fibrillation (ROTEA study). J Am Soc Echocardiogr. 2011;24(9):1046–1055.

126. Krishnaswamy A, Patel NS, Ozkan A, et al. Planning left atrial appendage occlusion using cardiac multidetector computed tomography. Int J Cardiol. 2012;158(2):313–317.

127. Kaafarani M, Saw J, Daniels M, et al. Role of CT imaging in left atrial appendage occlusion for the WATCHMAN device. Cardiovasc Diagn Ther. 2020;10(1):45–58.

128. Hiratzka LF, Bakris GL, Beckman JA, et al. 2010 ACCF/AHA/AATS/ACR/ASA/SCA/SCAI/SIR/STS/SVM guidelines for the diagnosis and management of patients with thoracic aortic disease. Circulation. 2010;121(13):e266–e369.

129. Goldstein, SA, Evangelista, A, Abbara, A, et al. Multimodality imaging of diseases of the thoracic aorta in adults: from the American Society of Echocardiography and the European Association of Cardiovascular Imaging: endorsed by the Society of Cardiovascular Computed Tomography and Society for Cardiovascular Magnetic Resonance. J Am Soc Echocardiogr. 2015 28(2):119–182.

130. Rajiah P, Schoenhagen P, Mehta D, et al. Low-dose, wide-detector array thoracic aortic CT angiography using an iterative reconstruction technique results in improved image quality with lower noise and fewer artifacts. J Cardiovasc Comput Tomogr. 2012;6(3):205–213.

131. Bolen MA, Popovic ZB, Tandon N, Flamm SD, Schoenhagen P, Halliburton SS. Image quality, contrast enhancement, and radiation dose of ECG-triggered high-pitch CT versus non-ECG-triggered standard-pitch CT of the thoracoabdominal aorta. AJR Am J Roentgenol. 2012;198(4):931–938.

132. Schoenhagen, P, Roselli EE. Acute Aortic Syndromes. AME Publishing Company, Hong Kong, 2018. ISBN: 978-988-78920-5-2.

133. Ueda T, Chin A, Petrovitch I, Fleischmann D. A pictorial review of acute aortic syndrome: discriminating and overlapping features as revealed by ECG-gated multidetector-row CT angiography. Insights Imaging. 2012;3(6):561–571.

134. Erdheim J. Medionecrosis aortae idiopathica cystica. Virch Arch Pathol Anat. 1930;276:187–229.

135. Svensson LG, Labib SB, Eisenhauer AC, Butterly JR. Intimal tear without hematoma: an important variant of aortic dissection that can elude current imaging techniques. Circulation. 1999;99:1331–1336.

136. Chin AS, Willemink MJ, Kino A, et al. Acute limited intimal tears of the thoracic aorta. J Am Coll Cardiol. 2018;71(24):2773–2785.

137. Braverman AC. Aortic dissection: prompt diagnosis and emergency treatment are critical. Cleve Clin J Med. 2011;78(10):685–696.

138. DeBakey ME, Henly WS, Cooley DA, Morris GC, Jr., Crawford ES, Beall AC, Jr. Surgical management of dissecting aneurysms of the aorta. J Thorac Cardiovasc Surg. 1965;49:130–149.

139. Lombardi JV, Hughes GC, Appoo JJ, et al. Ann Society for Vascular Surgery (SVS) and Society of Thoracic Surgeons (STS) Reporting Standards for Type B Aortic Dissections. Thorac Surg. 2020;109(3):959–981.

140. Buckley O, Rybicki FJ, Gerson DS, et al. Imaging features of intramural hematoma of the aorta. Int J Cardiovasc Imaging. 2010;26(1):65–76.

141. Moral S, Cuéllar H, Avegliano G, et al. Clinical implications of focal intimal disruption in patients with type b intramural hematoma. J Am Coll Cardiol. 2017;69(1):28–39.

142. Wu MT, Wang YC, Huang YL, et al. Intramural blood pools accompanying aortic intramural hematoma: CT appearance and natural course. Radiology. 2011;258(3):705–713.

143. Kitai T, Kaji S, Yamamuro A, et al. Impact of new development of ulcer-like projection on clinical outcomes in patients with type B aortic dissection with closed and thrombosed false lumen. Circulation. 2010;122(11 Suppl):S74–S80.

144. Gruettner J, Fink C, Walter T, et al. Coronary computed tomography and triple rule out CT in patients with acute chest pain and an intermediate cardiac risk profile. Part 1: impact on patient management. Eur J Radiol. 2013;82(1):100–105.

145. Stillman AE, Oudkerk M, Ackerman M, et al. Use of multidetector computed tomography for the assessment of acute chest pain: a consensus statement of the North American Society of Cardiac Imaging and the European Society of Cardiac Radiology. Eur Radiol. 2007;17(8):2196–2207.

146. Kitai T, Kaji S, Yamamuro A, et al. Impact of new development of ulcer-like projection on clinical outcomes in patients with type B aortic dissection with closed and thrombosed false lumen. Circulation. 2010;122(11 Suppl):S74–S80.

147. Song JK, Yim JH, Ahn JM, et al. Outcomes of patients with acute type A aortic intramural hematoma. Circulation. 2009;120(21):2046–2052.

148. Uchida K, Imoto K, Karube N, et al. Intramural haematoma should be referred to as thrombosed-type aortic dissection. Eur J Cardiothorac Surg. 2013. [Epub ahead of print]

149. Harris KM, Braverman AC, Eagle KA, et al. Acute aortic intramural hematoma: an analysis from the International Registry of Acute Aortic Dissection. Circulation. 2012;126(11 Suppl 1):S91–S96.

150. Paravastu SC, Ghosh J, Murray D, Farquharson FG, Serracino-Inglott F, Walker MG. A systematic review of open versus endovascular repair of inflammatory abdominal aortic aneurysms. Eur J Vasc Endovasc Surg. 2009;38(3):291–297.

151. Parmer SS, Carpenter JP, Stavropoulos SW, et al. Endoleaks after endovascular repair of thoracic aortic aneurysms. J Vasc Surg. 2006;44:447–452.

152. Resch TA, Greenberg RK, Lyden SP, et al. Combined staged procedures for the treatment of thoracoabdominal aneurysms. J Endovasc Ther. 2006;13:481–489.

153. O'Neill S, Greenberg RK, Haddad F, Resch T, Sereika J, Katz E. A prospective analysis of fenestrated endovascular grafting: intermediate-term outcomes. Eur J Vasc Endovasc Surg. 2006;32:115–123.

154. Azizzadeh A, Estrera AL, Porat EE, Madsen KR, Safi HJ. The hybrid elephant trunk procedure: a single-stage repair of an ascending, arch, and descending thoracic aortic aneurysm. J Vasc Surg. 2006;44:404–407.

155. Kamdar AR, Meadows TA, Roselli EE, et al. Multidetector computed tomographic angiography in planning of reoperative cardiothoracic surgery. Ann Thorac Surg. 2008;85(4):1239–1245.

156. To AC, Schoenhagen P, Desai MY. Role of tomographic imaging in preoperative planning and postoperative assessment in cardiovascular surgery. Heart. 2013. [Epub ahead of print] No abstract available.

157. Macleod MR, Amarenco P, Davis SM, Donnan GA. Atheroma of the aortic arch: an important and poorly recognised factor in the aetiology of stroke. Lancet Neurol. 2004;3:408–414.

158. Kurra V, Lieber ML, Sola S, et al. Extent of thoracic aortic atheroma burden and long-term mortality after cardiothoracic surgery: a computed tomography study. JACC Cardiovasc Imaging. 2010;3(10):1020–1029.

159. Aghayev A, Bay CP, Tedeschi S, et al. Clinically isolated aortitis: imaging features and clinical outcomes: comparison with giant cell arteritis and giant cell aortitis. Int J Cardiovasc Imaging. 2021 Apr;37(4):1433–1443. Epub 2020 Oct 30.

160. Chowdhary VR, Crowson CS, Bhagra AS, Warrington KJ, Vrtiska TJ. CT angiographic imaging characteristics of thoracic idiopathic aortitis. J Cardiovasc Comput Tomogr. 2013;7(5):297–302. Epub 2013 Sep 26.

161. Fleischmann D, Lammer J. Peripheral CT angiography for interventional treatment planning. Eur Radiol. 2006;16 Suppl 7:M58–M64.

162. Schernthaner R, Stadler A, Lomoschitz F, et al. Multidetector CT angiography in the assessment of peripheral arterial occlusive disease: accuracy in detecting the severity, number, and length of stenoses. Eur Radiol. 2008;18:665–671.

163. Fleischmann D, Rubin GD. Quantification of intravenously administered contrast medium transit through the peripheral arteries: implications for CT angiography. Radiology. 2005;236:1076–1082.

164. Roos JE, Fleischmann D, Koechl A, et al. Multipath curved planar reformation of the peripheral arterial tree in CT angiography. Radiology. 2007;244:281–290.

165. Met R, Bipat S, Legemate DA, Reekers JA, Koelemay MJ. Diagnostic performance of computed tomography angiography in peripheral arterial disease: a systematic review and meta-analysis. JAMA. 2009;301:415–424.

166. Ouwendijk R, de Vries M, Pattynama PM, et al. Imaging peripheral arterial disease: a randomized controlled trial comparing contrast-enhanced MR angiography and multi-detector row CT angiography. Radiology. 2005;236:1094–1103.

167. Schernthaner R, Fleischmann D, Stadler A, Schernthaner M, Lammer J, Loewe C. Value of MDCT angiography in developing treatment strategies for critical limb ischemia. AJR Am J Roentgenol. 2009;192:1416–1424.

168. Kau T, Eicher W, Reiterer C, et al. Dual-energy CT angiography in peripheral arterial occlusive disease-accuracy of maximum intensity projections in clinical routine and subgroup analysis. Eur Radiol. 2011;21:1677–1686.

169. Prakash P, Kalra MK, Stone JR, Shepard JA, Digumarthy SR. Imaging findings of pericardial metastasis on chest computed tomography. J Comput Assist Tomogr. 2010;34(4):554–558.

170. Hoey E, Ganeshan A, Nader K, Randhawa K, Watkin R. Cardiac neoplasms and pseudotumors: imaging findings on multidetector CT angiography. Diagn Interv Radiol. 2012;18(1):67–77.

171. Rajiah P, Kanne JP, Kalahasti V, Schoenhagen P. Computed tomography of cardiac and pericardiac masses. J Cardiovasc Comput Tomogr. 2011;5(1):16–29.

172. Anavekar NS, Bonnichsen CR, Foley TA, et al. Computed tomography of cardiac pseudotumors and neoplasms. Radiol Clin North Am. 2010;48(4):799–816.

173. Han BK, Rigsby CK, Hlavacek A, et al; Society of Cardiovascular Computed Tomography; Society of Pediatric Radiology; North American Society of Cardiac Imaging. Computed Tomography Imaging in Patients with Congenital Heart Disease Part I: Rationale and Utility. An Expert Consensus Document of the Society of Cardiovascular Computed Tomography (SCCT): Endorsed by the Society of Pediatric Radiology (SPR) and the North American Society of Cardiac Imaging (NASCI). J Cardiovasc Comput Tomogr. 2015;9(6):475–492. Epub 2015 Jul 23.

174. Han BK, Rigsby CK, Leipsic J, et al; Society of Cardiovascular Computed Tomography; Society of Pediatric Radiology; North American Society of Cardiac Imaging. Computed tomography imaging in patients with congenital heart disease, Part 2: Technical recommendations. An expert consensus document of the Society of Cardiovascular Computed Tomography (SCCT): endorsed by the Society of Pediatric Radiology (SPR) and the North American Society of Cardiac Imaging (NASCI). J Cardiovasc Comput Tomogr. 2015;9(6):493–513. Epub 2015 Aug 28.

175. Bartel T, Müller S. Contemporary echocardiographic guiding tools for device closure of interatrial communications. Cardiovasc Diagn Ther. 2013;3(1):38–46.

176. Gurudevan SV, Shah H, Tolstrup K, Siegel R, Krishnan SC. Septal thrombus in the left atrium: is the left atrial septal pouch the culprit? JACC Cardiovasc Imaging. 2010;3(12):1284–1286.

177. Tugcu A, Okajima K, Jin Z, et al. Septal pouch in the left atrium and risk of ischemic stroke. JACC Cardiovasc Imaging. 2010;3(12):1276–1283.

178. Angelini P, Velasco JA, Flamm S. Coronary anomalies: incidence, pathophysiology, and clinical relevance. Circulation. 2002;105(20):2449–2454.

179. Krasuski RA, Magyar D, Hart S, et al. Long-term outcome and impact of surgery on adults with coronary arteries originating from the opposite coronary cusp. Circulation. 2011;123(2):154–162.

180. Cremer PC, Mentias A, Koneru S, et al. Risk stratification with exercise N(13)-ammonia PET in adults with anomalous right coronary arteries. Open Heart. 2016;3(2):e000490. eCollection 2016.

Index

Note: Locators in *italics* represent figures in the text.